MW01065413

POTLUCK SURVIVAL GUIDE

Care and Feeding of the Athletic Supporter

• • • by Cherie Kimmons • • •

Five Star Publications, Inc.
Chandler, AZ

Linda F. Radke, President

Five Star Publications, Inc.

PO Box 6698

Chandler, AZ 85246-6698

480-940-8182

www.PotluckSurvivalGuide.com

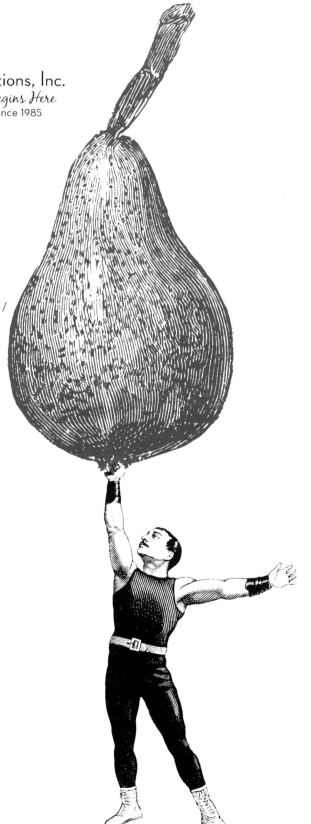

Library of Congress Cataloging-in-Publication Data

Kimmons, Cherie.
 Potluck survival guide : the care and feeding of the athletic supporter /
by Cherie Kimmons. -- 1st ed.
    p. cm.
 ISBN-13: 978-1-58985-073-6
 ISBN-10: 1-58985-073-4
 1. Cookery, American. 2. Athletes--Nutrition. 3. Youth--Nutrition. I.
Title.
 TX715.K49925 2008
 641.5973--dc22

                        2008017444

Printed in Canada

Cover design by Linda Longmire
Interior design by Linda Longmire
Indexing by Janet Bergin
Project Manager Sue DeFabis

TABLE OF CONTENTS

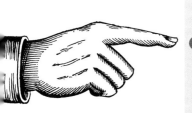

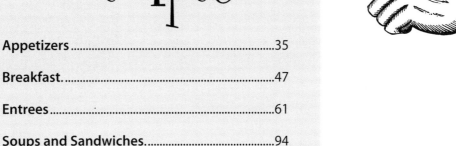

• • • Recipes • • •

Acknowledgments

THIS BOOK HAS BEEN A LABOR – sometimes of love, often of frustration. I never would have started it if my publisher, Linda Radke, hadn't, when she first heard my idea, said "I want that book!" Her support for this project inspired me.

Additionally, I want to thank all the gracious women – and men! – who contributed to this book without hesitation. I could not have attempted this book without their generous sharing of recipes and encouragement. A special thanks to Sheron Bibee, Patti Pearson, Cindy Baird and Kathy Hall, who shared their recipes as well as their wonderful decorating ideas. Leah Moir also was a boon and blessing, especially since she not only contributed recipes but listened to my uninterrupted moaning and groaning about the book on a regular basis.

My precious daughter, Emily, gave me invaluable editorial feedback from the viewpoint of a novice cook, as well as unrelenting enthusiasm and sympathy. My son, Patrick, loaned his taste buds and stomach during the long recipe testing process. The child will – and did! – eat anything, and had some pretty sophisticated suggestions for improving recipes.

And sweet Kim, my long-suffering husband and a handy cook in his own right, never once complained and never once doubted I would one day finish. He has come a long way from the man I married who was terrified of tamale pie. He is my favorite entrée.

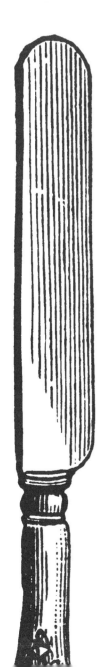
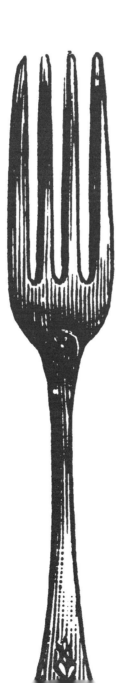
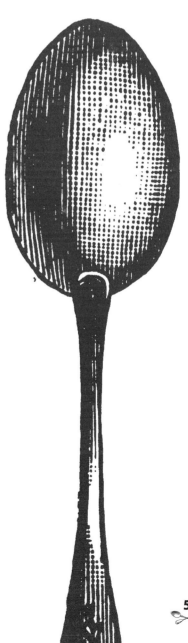

Pre-Game: Introduction

W e've all been there: you get the call one evening asking you to bring a dish to your school or church's next potluck. You panic. You want to take something that will impress the adults and have them begging for the recipe. You want the kids to come back for seconds so you don't go home with a half-full dish of food that you'll be eating for the next three days. But you don't want to spend a fortune on ingredients and hours in the kitchen using every pot and pan in the house. You especially don't want to show up with some generic-tasting food in a plastic container you nabbed at the grocery store on the way to the event (although you have gotten away with putting Chips Ahoy on a fancy plate in the past). Most of all, you just don't know what to fix.

So the process begins. You start your search in the mass of cookbooks that line your shelf. You find recipes for liver pate and ice cream towers surrounded with puff pastry. Nope. You love the recipe for a chicken dish until you notice it requires something described as the "tender part of lemon grass." What? Or how about that one that uses dried porcini mushrooms refreshed in a wine bath? Yikes! You have all these cookbooks, but can find only a few recipes that will work for your potluck drama. It's like owning a CD with only three tracks you like.

Brothers and sisters, I feel your pain. I have spent many nights reading my cookbooks in bed, trying to figure out what to fix – quick before I fall asleep. I have scanned the newspaper like a secret agent looking for hidden clues, searching for recipes that might be good for feeding crowds, feeding kids, or feeding crowds of kids. I've been at it for years.

Enough! I finally did what I wish someone had done for me years ago: collected all the recipes that work for feeding kids and their families and put them into a single book. That means just one volume on the bedside table, not a dangerous pile of twenty.

I have two children, now grown, who played sports all during their school years. I have cleaned uniforms for lacrosse, soccer, basketball, football, and baseball - plus ballet and horseback riding, which don't have uniforms, actually, but do produce lots of laundry.

I've spent roughly twenty years as a team-mom, room mother, food committee member and senior lunch chair; I've seen the good, the bad and the unappetizing on a buffet table. I've had a chance to see what kids will eat, and what they run from.

I've fed boys before the game and after the game; I've fed parents and visiting teams at double-headers; I've supplied the concession stand and the bake sales. I've helped feed teachers at Appreciation Lunches. I've helped feed parents at team meetings. I've fed lunch to senior classes. In short, I've learned how to feed a lot of people for a lot of different reasons. And, I've made all the mistakes so you don't have to (don't mix young kids with artichoke hearts).

Through the years, I have amassed a collection of recipes, begging them from other mothers, clipping them from magazines and newspapers, and gathering them from relatives and friends. Often, their origins are murky, coming from scribbles on the back of an envelope. Some seem to have been around since the dawn of time. Through the years I've honed these recipes, making them crowd- or kid-friendly.

I come from a long line of exceptional cooks, and I inherited their affinity for spices and experimentation. My mother hit the culinary jackpot with an Italian father and Cajun French mother. She grew up eating food that was simple and intensely flavored, like smoky gumbo, venison marinated in mustard and garlic, snapper stuffed with crab or eggplant, a chicken from the back yard fried up fresh, or fragrant hot loaves of "old lady face bread" covered in pepper and garlic. Food was cause for celebration and, on Sundays, a nap.

Mom learned early on how to use any and every ingredient that crossed her path. During her big cooking years, her refrigerator was a forest of recycled jars bearing a masking tape label: leftover gravy, cooking water from Sunday's corned beef, a little hollandaise here, a bit of honey mustard there. Somehow, all those things found new life in another dish. Nothing (nothing!) was ever thrown away. She frequently flew without a net, creating unique, unreproducible concoctions with her little cache of secret ingredients on the refrigerator shelves. Her perfect vegetable soup has never been the same twice. It always is fabulous. It is in this book.

Here are the recipes that you can go to any time you need ideas for feeding kids, ball teams, parents, teachers, scouts, the book club, or tailgaters. These are recipes that work, that are tried-and-true favorites of young and old alike.

They are not wild experimental forays into flavored foams. You won't find cutting-edge ingredient combinations, or complicated techniques. Many of the recipes contain ingredients that will never appear on the table of a five-star restaurant, like canned soup and Velveeta cheese (which, by the way, has its own dictionary entry). But these simple ingredients often are what make a dish children enjoy. Think comfort food; think home-cooking. Whatever is in them, they are the most requested recipes at any party they attend.

Are these recipes all healthy and diet conscious? Well, yes and no. Some recipes are not meant to be light. Brownies, the number one favorite dessert of school children everywhere, are best eaten in their full, chocolaty, buttery glory. Macaroni and cheese is just sad made with a quarter cup of low-fat cheese and skim milk. You won't find the youngsters lining up for that one. One of the reasons some of the recipes are so popular with the kids is because they do have lots of cheese, sugar, or whipping cream. You can't fight that.

The good news is many of the recipes can be prepared several ways. When suitable, a recipe will include a healthy variation, using lighter options or lower fat. In some cases, suggestions for sneaking in vegetables are included. Keep in mind, however, that the original recipe is usually the one that lines 'em up at the dinner table.

Other recipes are healthy from the git-go. While younger children might not be interested in a crisp string bean, many teens are definitely health-conscious. The popularity of salad has never been higher. When my eldest was young, the only person eating salad at the buffet table was the sad-eyed woman trying to lose weight. Now, salad is the only thing many teen-aged girls will eat at a school buffet. The salad bowl is usually empty by the end of the night, no matter what the occasion is. Whether people are trying to eat healthy, or trying to feel better about taking so much macaroni and cheese, they are eating salad. No longer a wallflower at these events, the salad bowl has become a main attraction.

Some recipes also have a vegetarian option, while others have a note when meat can be added to transform it from a side dish into an entrée. Most recipes will have suggestions for optional seasonings and additions. Ways to make a recipe kid-friendly (don't add those green olives!) or more adult-appropriate (perhaps a bit of blue cheese?) are included. Recipes especially favored by children will be noted.

I also have included some "master recipes" that go into great detail explaining the ingredients and methods used in the preparation of a basic dish, like mashed potatoes and boiled chicken. A security blanket for novice cooks and, perhaps, a refresher course for the more experienced cook, these master recipes are the building blocks for countless variations. My hope is that they will provide enough information about the whys and hows of a recipe that you will feel comfortable enough to begin to experiment, really making the recipe your own.

One of the goals of this book is to help you match the needs of your crowd to your menu. The experience of feeding athletes and their families is what inspired this book, and athletes have special needs. Appropriate food for athletes before a game is very different from what they want to eat on the bus ride home. Nervous stomachs and nutritional considerations are critical to menu choices. You will find information for the proper care and feeding of young athletes before a game, along with tips from coaches and suggestions for post-game food when you are playing away from home.

You can benefit from the mistakes I made in this area. I once sent a platter of sliced tomatoes and shredded lettuce on the team bus for the ride home. It was to be used for discretionary placement on post-game sandwiches. The boys were too wound up after the game for so much loose food. Coach informed me that vegetable Frisbees and lettuce confetti made the ride home seem a whole lot longer than usual. I was a happier person before knowing these things. I am a wiser one now.

Another goal of this book is to take the fear out of feeding kids about whom you may know nothing in the way of food preferences. There is a section with tips and hints for feeding kids in ways that will result in food actually being eaten.

A big part of feeding a team during the school years is decorating the eating space. If you are lucky enough to be involved with a sport that has cheerleaders, you are practically home free; the cheerleaders will be a huge help. I strongly suspect they have to pass a magic-marker and butcher paper competency test to make the squad.

But never fear. If you are going solo in the decorating department, I have information just for you. I have worked with some remarkably creative women over the years and they have shared their decorating secrets with me. They've helped me amass lots of easy and inexpensive ideas for transforming the cafeteria or game-side tabletops. Who could resist a lovely, fresh flower arrangement in a baseball cup? Or cap? Both are pretty cheap.

If you are stuck with planning an entire meal for a large group, flip to the chapter with a chart for estimating the quantities of ingredients you will need. Then just multiply how many batches of a recipe you'll need and start delegating. You will also find suggestions for menus for different occasions and for different diners. And my favorite chapter is the Hall of Fame Recipes that lists a few of the best recipes in this book. If you can only fix one or two recipes from this book, try one of these.

I have learned through the years that quality counts in cooking. Your dish will be no better that the ingredients you use. Remember that old computer term, garbage in - garbage out? Well, it applies here, too. No matter how perfect the recipe, if you don't use good ingredients, you won't get good results. For the best-tasting dishes, you need to use the freshest food you can find. This is especially true for simple preparations, where each ingredient becomes critically important to the final result. Don't use the garlic that has started growing green tips, or carrots that sag.

I have discovered some wonderful sources for ingredients that I use regularly. In the Recruiting chapter, you will find a list of these resources for some of the highest quality ingredients available. I urge you to try some of these remarkable purveyors. You might be shocked at the difference truly fresh chili powder makes in your tamale pie!

So jump in! You might find a few of your old favorite recipes that have been floating around for years. I hope you'll find some new favorites that you can't wait to try at the next team picnic or Sunday lunch.

GAME Plan: FIGURING OUT THE MENU

Okay. So what do you do when your worst nightmare comes true? You don't just have to think of one dish to take to a potluck – you have to think of a dish for everyone to bring. You are in charge of the whole shebang, or at least figuring out a menu and delegating cooking chores. Probably, if you are the designated decision maker, you got there through merit. You have a gift for organization that was recognized by higher powers (or else you were in the bathroom when they took a vote for committee chairperson). If you are not gifted with the organization gene, but you have to organize the event anyway, don't panic. You can work your way through this and survive.

Designing a menu requires a little thought. It helps to have some structure. The following guidelines are a good starting point in designing a balanced meal.

- **Balance appearance:** have different colors and textures to make a pretty plate. Chicken, served with mashed potatoes, cauliflower and a pale iceberg lettuce salad may taste wonderful, but the eye goes hungry (or just as bad, gets bored). This is where colorful vegetables and fruits can save the day. A little steamed broccoli or green beans, a slice of tomato, or a mixed fruit salad would be colorful companions to the chicken. Garnishes go a long way toward adding a little colorful zing. A ruffle of parsley on a meat platter, a cherry red tomato in the midst of something brown or green, a lettuce bed for the deviled eggs – it doesn't take much to make it pretty. The bonus is the good nutrition that usually accompanies all those different-colored foods.

- **Balance weight:** coordinate the dessert and entrée. If the entrée is a simple, feeds-a-lot-for-cheap recipe, have a spectacular dessert. Soup and grilled cheese sandwiches would benefit from a slab of dangerous chocolate cake. If your entrée is killer, end with a lighter dessert, like fruit or cookies. Cheesecake would be redundant with a rich or elaborate entrée, like crab strata, or brisket and mashed potatoes. Pull out the baked fruit recipes and top them with a little oatmeal and sugar, or dizzy them up with a splash of brandy.

- **Balance techniques:** don't use the same technique for every dish. The main culprit here is frying –you don't want to have fried chicken, French fries and fried pies on your menu – unless your theme is cardiac surgery. (Besides – all that brown food needs more color!) The exception to this rule might be a New England boiled dinner, or corned beef and cabbage – more a one-pot meal than repetition of a technique.

- **Balance flavors:** don't use the same, strong-flavored, distinctive ingredient in multiple dishes. Blue cheese needs to appear only once, as do jalapenos and tomatoes (unless you have a Mexican theme going). If you are serving spaghetti with marinara sauce, you don't want a pasta salad side dish or stewed tomatoes and okra. The bottom line is variety in color, taste, and texture.

The most important aspect of the job ahead of you is actually to feed the crowd. You will need to know who your audience is. Who are you feeding? Young kids? Athletes? Teenagers? Parents? The age of your group will influence your food choices. As a rule, younger children like plainer food, while adults generally are more flexible and adventuresome (even if you are feeding a crowd of adults, it is wise to steer clear of really radical recipes when feeding a crowd). Just what does it take to get young kids interested in the meal?

• • • FEEDING CHILDREN • • •

If the event you are planning involves school or a sports team, you might have little mouths to feed. This can be challenging; young kids are notoriously picky eaters. Of course, every rule has its exception. Somewhere, there is a five-year-old whose favorite dish is a truffle omelet. Some kids are exposed to sophisticated flavors early in their eating careers and love olives and bright green food, but you are safer playing to the lowest common denominator when menu planning for the little guys. The truffle kid is more likely to happily wolf down mac and cheese than the timid guy is to try the mushroom casserole.

Let's look at some of the considerations that affect menu choices for feeding young children, around the ages of 5 to 10 years, well as some considerations for feeding their older brothers and sisters. Please keep in mind these are generalizations.

- One of the most important things to remember if you are feeding young kids is is to **KEEP IT SIMPLE**. Young kids don't get excited over a lot of choices; they get excited about lots of the stuff they like. You don't need tremendous variety; fewer dishes are actually better for younger kids so they won't be overwhelmed with too many choices. And, it is easier for you! Just make sure the few dishes you do present are top-notch.

- **Skip fancy** – don't use recipes with elaborate sauces, unusual or highly spiced flavors, or scary-looking vegetables (this would include eggplant in any shape or form). Usually you can modify most recipes to suit younger children by eliminating highly flavored or colored ingredients like green and black olives, green onions and green peppers, (whether in the dish or used as a garnish.) Parsley is just a waste of good money for this age group. Look for flavors that are uncomplicated; think Velveeta cheese.

- Young children like to be able to identify their food; casseroles can be traumatizing for a child who is used to food arriving in styrofoam containers at the drive-thru. **Serve young children food that looks like what it is**. Some of the most popular menus for young children mimic fast food offerings: sausage and biscuits, chicken sandwiches (minus lettuce and tomato, of course), pizza or tacos. Your "touch" for these common foods will be using excellent ingredients. Leave exploration of new flavors to the family table. This is not the time to spring an exotic dish on young diners unless you just really like having lots of leftovers and cranky, hungry children.

- **Healthy is not impossible**, sometimes it just requires stealth. If you are serving sandwiches, make them on light-colored whole wheat bread. If you have a sauce for spaghetti, chop the veggies really fine and no one will ever know they are in there. Opt for leaner cuts of meat when possible. In line with keeping it simple, just don't give kids an unhealthy choice. If there is no chip alternative, kids will dig in to veggie sticks or fruit kebabs. Hunger is a wonderful thing.

- As kids get older, **salads become a viable option**. With younger children, keep the lettuce simple: romaine is a good choice –flavorful and more nutritious than iceberg. With older children, you can use more diverse varieties. Pre-washed and bagged baby lettuces are great - pretty, flavorful, and so easy. Check the food club in your neighborhood for large quantities of cleaned mixed lettuces.

- You can also tempt kids to eat a little salad if there are **fun things to put on top**: cheese, bacon, croutons, dressing choices. If you are serving salad on a buffet line, combine the basic salad ingredients – lettuce, cucumbers, carrot shreds, tomatoes, e.g., – in a large bowl and arrange the fun/exotic toppings on the side. A child who would pass up a salad with visible olives and green peppers might put a little on the plate if it was only lettuce and there is a bottle of Ranch nearby. Ranch dressing is the number one favorite dressing of kids of all ages. You would be surprised what kids will dip in Ranch dressing. Surprised and disgusted. Have regular and light versions available, especially if you are serving teenagers.

- **Watch the nuts** – a lot of kids don't like them, and there is always one in the crowd who is allergic to them. If you are going to serve nuts (and here I am referring to the food, not the kids), make sure the dish is labeled.

- Kids of all ages like **things they can hold in their hands**; forks and knives are for the civilized. Kids are more likely to pick up and eat something they can carry away in their hands without a plate. Sandwiches, tacos, a piece of fried chicken, a sausage biscuit – all are good walking-around food. Older kids are attracted to carry-around food, too. Especially dessert. Favorite desserts include highly transportable cookies, brownies, and cake cut into small, non-toppling squares. Brownies are the number one favorite kid dessert. Chocolate that doesn't need a plate - perfect!

- In the same vein, cut up fresh fruit or vegetables into **bite-sized pieces**. Don't serve a whole orange; segments will move a lot faster – kids will just grab one or two and keep moving. Instead of a whole apple, slice it – and maybe slather on some peanut butter to up the ante.

- Around twelve or thirteen, a lot of kids go through a vegetarian phase, and more and more adults are foregoing meat these days. Although vegetarians are practiced at finding food they can consume in this meat-eating world, always try to **have at least one dish a vegetarian can eat**. This will often be a hearty side dish. Sometimes just adding cheese will make a vegetable dish suitable as a main dish for a vegetarian. Consider adding cheese to your sides when appropriate. You can also offer two versions of the same dish: chili with meat and without, cheese pizza and pepperoni pizza, a breakfast casserole with and without sausage.

- As a rule, **younger kids don't enjoy potato salad**, a potluck staple. There are so many unknown things swimming around in that mayonnaise. **Try deviled eggs instead**. They don't require a fork, which gives them a certain charm, and they are full of high-quality protein. Potato salad is no problem for older kids, and deviled eggs seem to be a favorite with males of any age. At the buffet table, they are one of the first things to go

- As mentioned earlier, younger kids seem to like **food that is familiar**, which, in their case, is fast food. Hamburgers, chicken, pizza, biscuits, tacos – those are all safe choices to serve the younger set. While a meal of pizza might seem mundane to you, to young kids it borders on exciting. On the other hand, older kids seem to go for the **home-cooked taste**. They have had plenty of experience with fast food and cafeteria food and they like something that tastes like home: brisket and mashed potatoes, chicken and dressing casserole (a perennial favorite), vegetable soup and grilled cheese sandwiches.

- You don't have to fulfill all the health requirements for the entire day in one meal. **Offer healthy choices and reasonable variety**, and let the chips (or veggie sticks) fall where they may. Accept that some kids will not like some of what is offered. They will not starve to death if they don't take a full plate, or leave most of the food uneaten. They will make up for it at the next meal. And no one died from eating all desserts at one meal. I am living proof.

- Don't feel you always have to do the cooking yourself. **Have a favorite restaurant cater** a particular item that is especially popular with the kids. You don't have to have the whole meal catered, just those popular items, whether it's pounds of barbecue or fried chicken sandwiches. A local Italian restaurant in my town makes fabulous garlic rolls the kids love; several large pans of the rolls are easy to pre-order and pick up on meal day. Ditto bacon – a restaurant can fry up several pounds for pick-up, and they have to deal with all the grease, not you. This is a great option for working parents who might not have extra time to spend in the kitchen.

• • • Kid-friendly Menus • • •

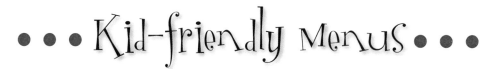

Remember that young children like fast food and simple ingredients. These menus have uncomplicated flavors and don't offer too many choices.

Sausage Links rolled in Pancakes/Syrup Baked Fruit	Fried chicken Company potatoes Green beans Chocolate Chip Treasure Cookies
Sausage and biscuit sandwiches Fresh fruit Yogurt with granola	Sloppy Joes Mac and cheese Carrot and celery sticks with Ranch dressing for dipping Texas Sheet Cake
Healthy muffins Crisp bacon Fruit Kebab - fresh fruit on a skewer with yogurt dipping sauce	Chicken Noodle Soup Pimento cheese sandwiches Cut fresh fruit Sugar cookies
Pizza Sandwiches (easier to handle than floppy pizza slices) OR Stromboli Fruit Kebabs with yogurt dipping sauce Ice Cream Sandwich Cake	Mini Empanadas Mixed salad and dressing Corn pudding Enhanced chocolate chip cookies
Hot Dogs Deluxe Baked Beans Veggie sticks and Ranch dressing No-bake chocolate oatmeal cookies	

••• Kid-friendly Recipes •••

These recipes are appropriate for and popular with kids of any age. The ingredient list is fairly short and often includes Velveeta cheese and canned soup. Some of these dishes are blander than what I would serve at an all-adult meal, but they can be jazzed up for any palate with the addition of stronger flavors, perhaps a sharp cheddar cheese instead of Velveeta. But note that many adults love the simple flavors of these uncomplicated dishes, too. I have only listed entrees and sides – kids generally don't have much trouble with dessert of any sort – well, unless it has visible raisins. If you need a dish for a church or school event that includes younger kids, just scan these.

Entrees	Sides and Salad
Basic Beef Noodle Casserole	Baked Fruit
Casserole Spaghetti	Overnight Company Potatoes
Chicken Noodle Soup	Cornbread casserole
Cow-puncher Beef and Rice	Corn Pudding
Ham Delights	Fried Bread
Hot Dogs Deluxe	Favorite Green Beans
King Ranch Casserole	Hash Brown Casserole
Layered Hamburger Casserole	Mandarin Salad
Mini Empanadas	Nana's Baked Beans
Mom's Pimento Cheese	Old-fashioned Mac and Cheese
Nana's Garlic Brisket	Overnight Company Potatoes
Pizza Sandwiches	
Potato and Egg Bake	
Sausage Cheese Muffins	
Sausage Mac and Cheese	
Sloppy Joes	
Stromboli	
Tagliarini	
Texas Shepherd Pie	
Thanksgiving Casserole	

••• Feeding Athletes •••

When you have athletes to keep fed and hydrated, the rules for menu planning change a bit. If you are in charge of feeding a team before, during, or after a game, you have a whole new set of considerations. Always check with the coach for guidelines before planning a meal for athletes. Your main concern is not going to be how the food tastes; food becomes fuel in an athletic setting, and you have to figure out which octane to use. You must take into account what the food is (fat, carbohydrate, or protein), and when it is eaten.

First, let's talk about the "what." All the coaches with whom I've worked in the past and most current health gurus agree: carbohydrates are the most important component in a meal before a game or practice. Remember "carb loading" from years ago? This is it. Carbs are easy to digest, so their calories are quickly available as fuel. They don't sit heavy in a nervous stomach, the way fat and protein can.

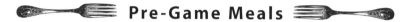 **Pre-Game Meals**

The USA Swimming organization is a group that has an athlete's nutrition down to a fine art. Swimmers are especially sensitive to the issue of pre-game and workout meals. The group's website suggests each of the following meals to provide 100 grams of carbohydrates as an appropriate pre-game meal:

> ### PRE-GAME MEALS WITH 100 GRAMS OF CARBOHYDRATES
>
> • 1 bagel with peanut butter and 2/3 cup of raisins
>
> • 1 cup low-fat yogurt, 1 banana and 1 cup of orange juice
>
> • 1 turkey sandwich with 1 cup applesauce
>
> • 2 cups of spaghetti with meat sauce and 1 piece of garlic bread
>
> • 8 ounces of skim milk, 1 apple, 1 orange, 2 slices of bread and 3 pancakes
>
> • 1 serving of Gatorade and 1 bagel

You get the idea: light on the protein, heavy on the carb-y food like pasta, bread and fruit. Fortunately, these foods are portable and easy to pack in your trunk or find at a fast food restaurant. Turkey sandwiches were the fall-back choice for pre-game and between-game meals on a hot day for my son's baseball team. The boys were sick of Subway sandwiches by the end of the season, but they learned the hard way that chili dogs were not a good choice. (There is always one kid in the crowd who can eat nachos with extra jalapenos in 98-degree heat and never feel a thing, but it isn't a good idea for the majority of kids.)

Timing is the other critical food factor for athletes. On game day, several small meals with an emphasis on carbs are preferable to one huge feeding before an event. These small, regular doses of food keep the blood sugar levels stable. Fat and protein should be eaten at times that are not close to a workout or game. Generally, two hours is considered a good window of time before a game for heavier food.

For you football parents, the pre-game meal usually occurs more than two hours before the game, so these restrictions are not as important. Balanced and healthy should be the focus for the pre-game meal, as well as variety. Try to have offerings that accommodate different levels of nervousness. A full course meal with meat, sides, salad and dessert is a fine starting point, but you should also include some choices for those who aren't comfortable eating heavily (even two hours) before a game. Some great offerings include yogurt, peanut butter and jelly sandwiches (be on the alert for nut allergies – we let the boys make their own sandwiches if they didn't go through the buffet line, so we weren't too concerned that a kid with allergies would make himself a PB&J), and milk and cereal. Fresh fruit is also appropriate. Bananas, apples or applesauce, and orange juice are good fuel foods that are easily tolerated.

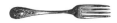 # Post Game Meals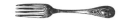

The most important time to eat, according to USAS, is in the first 30 minutes after practice or major physical exertion, and the offerings should include both carbs and protein to restore fuel stores and repair muscle tissue. For maximum recovery, a full meal should be eaten within two hours after practice or a game. This makes bus food really important for those away games and meets.

Fluid levels are also important. Make sure your child has plenty to drink during a meet or game. Usually, the coach will make sure players have access to fluid, but if you are the responsible party, be sure your child has several bottles of water. If the event lasts more than 90 minutes, include a sports drink, too. Avoid carbonated and caffeinated drinks. Caffeine contributes to fluid loss, and carbonation can cause bloating, which may reduce fluid intake, not to mention creating funky discomfort for your players.

IN A NUTSHELL: GUIDELINES FOR FEEDING ATHLETES

1. Pre-game meals should be heavy on carbs, light on protein and fat.

2. Allow 2 hours between a meal (especially a heavy one) and athletic event.

3. Feed athletes within 30 minutes after a major exertion to replenish their fuel stores.

4. A full-scale meal should be eaten within 2 hours after a major exertion for maximum muscle recovery and should include protein and carbohydrates.

5. Fluids during exertion are critical – 2 bottles of water are a minimum for a game. Avoid caffeine and carbonation.

6. If an event exceeds 90 minutes, include a sports drink in addition to the water.

Meals for Athletes

Based on the guidelines discussed above, here are some suggestions for getting fuel into your player. Fast food is not necessarily a poor option; in fact, for breakfast, fast food pancakes are quick and easy and usually enjoyed by most kids (especially the syrup).

 Breakfast
- Pancakes, waffles, French toast, bagels, cereal, English muffins, bran muffins
- Syrup and jam
- Light protein: scrambled eggs, yogurt, low-fat milk
- Fruit juices, fresh fruit, dried fruit
- **Avoid:** *sausage, bacon, fast-food breakfast sandwiches, butter*

 Lunch and Dinner
- Pastas, whole-grain bread, salad, baked potato
- Low-fat protein like turkey, low-fat cheese and yogurt
- Thick crust pizza - avoid high fat toppings like sausage, pepperoni and extra cheese
- Vegetable soup and chili with bread and crackers
- Fresh fruit and juice; fresh vegetables
- Low-fat milk shakes and frozen yogurt
- Emphasize bread in sandwiches, not the condiments
- Low-fat milk and fruit juice
- **Avoid:** *fried foods and carbonated drinks*

 Fast Food Restaurant Choices
- Chicken fajita
- Hamburger
- Broiled chicken sandwich
- Roast beef sandwich
- Bean burrito
- Cheese pizza
- Baked potato with chili
- Low-fat milkshakes
- Salads, either main dish or side

Bus food

Are the kids eating before the game or after? These are some good choices for pre-game meals or after school before practice begins.

Pre-Event

- Cheese Pizza
- Pimento Cheese sandwiches
- Fruit - cut in slices and put into individual servings in a plastic bag
- Pretzels – especially good pre-game since they are mild and salty to encourage fluid intake
- Clementine oranges – the kids love to peel and eat these (be prepared to find random pieces of peel for days)

- Grapes in zip top bags
- Nutty Cereal Snack
- Bagels/cream cheese – use the little bagels
- Little cups of yogurt
- Healthy muffins

Post-Event

After the game, win or lose, the ride home can seem long. Food helps fill the time and tummies. Your choices are wide open since you no longer need to worry about nervous guts and carb loading, but as noted above, it is important to replenish energy stores. Be sure to include plenty of liquids for dehydrated athletes. If you are playing away from home, consider ordering a slew of sandwiches from a local sandwich store for pick up or ordering pizza that can be delivered to the field.

- Sandwiches, homemade or from a sandwich store like Subway
- Roll-ups
- Stromboli
- Mini Empanadas

- Meatball sandwiches
- Brisket sandwiches
- Pizza of any flavor, delivered to the field before the bus leaves
- Chik-fil-A sandwiches

Trunk Food

If you need to feed kids on the run between school and practice, here are some ideas for portable meals you can keep in a cooler in the trunk or pick up along the way. During the season, you might want to keep a supply of moist towelettes, paper napkins or paper towels, and plastic cutlery tucked into the trunk, too. Try to keep the cleats and equipment separate from the food!

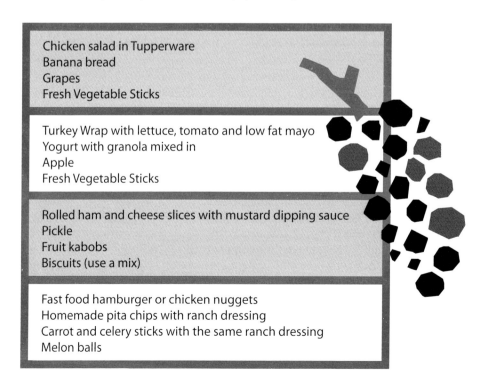

Chicken salad in Tupperware
Banana bread
Grapes
Fresh Vegetable Sticks

Turkey Wrap with lettuce, tomato and low fat mayo
Yogurt with granola mixed in
Apple
Fresh Vegetable Sticks

Rolled ham and cheese slices with mustard dipping sauce
Pickle
Fruit kabobs
Biscuits (use a mix)

Fast food hamburger or chicken nuggets
Homemade pita chips with ranch dressing
Carrot and celery sticks with the same ranch dressing
Melon balls

BuFFet StrateGies: Getting Food to the People

When you have to serve a crowd, the menu is the most obvious area of angst. Choosing what food to serve is fraught with multiple considerations including budget, audience, and wow factor. But an important consideration in deciding what to serve also involves, like good real estate, location, location, location. Where you serve the food is a critical feeding factor. If you are serving outside, you will need to think about keeping the food either warm or cold. The availability of electricity makes the job easy. Just don't forget an ample supply of extension cords.

Will you need to go the canned heat route? If you are stuck with canned heat, always have a few extra cans – more than you think you will need. If you are far from power lines, you may choose to serve food that sits well at room temperature and doesn't require a heat or cooling source. Fried chicken, ribs, cold cuts and sandwiches, salads and fruit, and nearly any (non-frozen) dessert work well under these conditions. If you have electricity (indoors or out), warming trays and slow cookers/crock pots are the amateur caterer's best friends. You can keep sandwiches warm in a crock pot as well as liquids and casseroles. If you are going to be involved in a lot of feeding events, you might want to consider investing in a warming tray; warming trays usually can accommodate several different shaped dishes easily (which is nice when you have potluck and so much variety in serving vessels). If you are serving a large crowd with people moving through rather quickly, you might want to use the warming trays to keep the food waiting in the wings warm. Place the hot dish on the serving table and as soon as it is empty, replace it with a dish from the warming tray. If food on the serving table is going to sit a while as diners drift through, use the warming trays on the table instead.

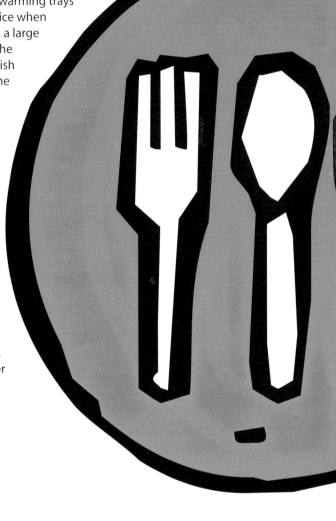

Keeping food cold is equally important. Coolers and ice are about the only way to go when you are serving outside. Get more ice than you think you need, and scrounge up as many coolers as you can – you will be surprised at how quickly they will be pressed into service. If you want to keep something cold on the serving table, you can rig up a two-layered arrangement. Start with an insulated container on the bottom and fill it with ice. Set the serving platter on top of the ice and hope for a cloudy day if you are serving outside. To make it look a little better, you could drape a pretty towel over the insulated bottom layer before setting the serving platter on it. If you are serving a ball team, don't bother with the pretty stuff – they are only interested in the calories.

Once you have designed your menu taking into consideration where it will be served, your next mission is to get the food to the people efficiently. Rather than setting up tables haphazardly and hoping for the best, consider some of these tips for organization and decoration:

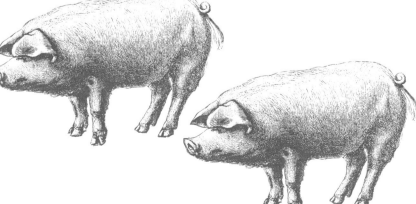

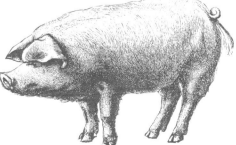

Buffet tips

- Try serving on **both sides of the table** for quicker processing. This means you will have to have doubles of everything, one for each side of the table. Be sure you have plenty of serving utensils.

- Place the dishes at the front end of the table, but leave the s**ilverware and napkins at the end** so folks don't have to juggle them while serving themselves in line.

- If you have the time and inclination, **wrap the cutlery in a napkin** for a quick, clean pickup by diners. Tuck the wrapped cutlery in a tall container. It helps prevent a slow-down at the end of the line.

- If you are in charge, always have a little emergency kit on hand: extra serving utensils – especially tongs and large spoons, a knife, tinfoil, plastic bags, masking tape, paper towels.

- Don't place the table near the front door, bathroom, or any other **high-traffic area**.

- Try to **set up the food in separate areas** to spread the crowd out – maybe separate beverage and dessert tables in addition to the entrée table.

- It is always a good idea to **label each dish**. It helps identify allergens or the presence of meat. It might also increase the likelihood that you won't have to carry home a pan full of food, since people are more likely to take something when they know what it is.

- For visual impact, **serve your food at different levels**, if possible. This is especially nice for dessert tables. If you don't have any fancy-schmancy pedestals, just cover boxes of different heights with cloth, either extra table cloths, napkins or fabric yardage. Tuck under raw edges. Set your serving pieces on top. All this extra fabric gives a luxurious, elegant look to the table. Just make sure you use fabric that can be washed or that won't be ruined with spills. This is a great opportunity to incorporate team colors or theme patterns.

- **Ice, ice, ice**. Have plenty of ice chests to keep the drinks cold. Have plenty of ice in the chests. Have more than you think you will need.

- Keeping beverages cold: if you are serving a punch, **freeze some of the liquid to use as ice cubes**. Freeze the liquid in regular ice cube trays, or maybe a round tube pan or coffee can if you will be serving from a large container. You can add cute little garnishes within each cube for a decorative touch. Try floating a raspberry or strawberry in fruit punch ice cubes, for example. Other options include rose petals, lime slices, mint leaves, even little slices of jalapeno.

- Freezing/re-heating: If you cook a casserole and then freeze it, check your original baking time in the recipe and **add 15 minutes to accommodate the colder temperature** of the dish. If the casserole is supposed to be covered for a portion of the usual baking time, leave the cover on for these extra 15 minutes before continuing to bake uncovered.

- Decorations: **fresh food makes an easy centerpiece** for the buffet table, piled in baskets or other containers. Grapes drape beautifully, and they can be sugar-frosted for a really festive look. Just mix a beaten egg white with a little bit of water and dip the grapes in the mixture. While they are still wet, roll them in granulated sugar and set on paper towels to dry.

- **Vegetables also look great in an arrangement**. Try grouping a lot of one item for impact. For example, fill a tall glass vase with artichokes, lemons or limes. Take a cue from your menu theme.

- **Squeeze bottles are good** for serving almost any condiment; they keep the food out of the air, they don't drip or require serving utensils, and kids think they are a blast to use. They are a lot faster to use in a line than a jar or dish and knife. Load them up with ketchup, mustard, mayonnaise, barbecue sauce, sour cream, chocolate or caramel sauce, creamy horseradish sauce, yogurt mixture for fruit, salad dressings, syrup – you get the idea! A label on the bottle is critical (try masking tape and a sharpie for a quick job of it). If you are putting a thicker liquid in the squeeze bottle, check to make sure the hole is big enough for the substance to come out quickly.

- Keep gravies and syrups warm in an **insulated carafe**. This makes pouring easier, too! Don't forget the label.

OPTION PLAY: The Food Bar

I f you are looking for a fun way to serve a lot of kids – or even regular people for that matter - try a "build-your-own" food bar. This concept has been popular with caterers and restaurants for years. Kids loving controlling what they put on their food, and they relish the choices. We all do!

Food bars work for a variety of foods from salad and entrees to desserts: baked potatoes, salad, tacos, chili, and sundaes. If you are setting up a food bar, use both sides of the table so diners can file down either side. This will speed up the service.

You might want to consider making labels for each topping. Use poster board or other stiff paper product. Cut the product into rectangles and fold in half so they make a stand-alone tent. Label one side. Or just use index cards folded in half and tented.

Baked Potato Bar

This is an easy, fun entrée to do. You can cook the potatoes in advance and keep them warm in crock pots. If this is a school event, check with your school cafeteria and see if they can prepare the potatoes for you. Large and small potatoes provide options for any size appetite. This is a good option for vegetarians, too. Here are some of the best-loved toppings:

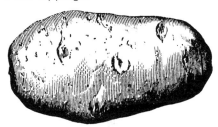

- Sour cream
- Butter
- Garlic butter
- Chopped green onions
- Chopped black olives
- Chopped steamed broccoli
- Chili (meat and/or bean)
- Shredded pork BBQ
- Sautéed veggies like mushrooms, onions, and peppers
- Cheddar cheese, shredded
- Crispy bacon bits
- Chives
- Sour cream French onion dip
- Jalapenos
- Blue cheese crumbles
- Browned and seasoned ground beef
- Ketchup (it's actually good – like eating French fries)
- Ranch dressing

Taco Bar

Tacos appeal to the masses. You can make a meat version and a bean version for vegetarians. For speedier service, you can pre-load the tacos with meat, or beans, or both and then let diners add their favorite toppings.

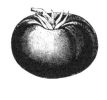

- Chopped tomatoes
- Chopped onions
- Black olives
- Guacamole
- Jalapenos
- Extra refried beans
- Chopped lettuce
- Chopped cilantro
- Salsa (hot and mild)
- Sour cream
- Shredded cheese

Chili Bar

This is a great one for the cold months, and easily pleases both vegetarians and meat eaters if you present meat and meatless versions (full of beans) of the chili. In the interest of expediency, you may want to have the chili already dished up and then let diners top their bowls with all the extras.

- Cheese
- Olives
- Oyster crackers
- Sour cream
- Cilantro
- Corn chips
- Chopped onions
- Jalapenos
- Extra beans (chili, black or kidney)
- Chopped tomatoes
- Fresh lime wedges

A variation on the chili bar is a nacho bar, using corn chips (either Frito-style, or Mexican-style chips) as a base. Pour on some chili and then start loading up the toppings. The kids seem to love the Fritos best under all those ingredients.

Salad Bar

This is the mack-daddy of food bars. A salad can become the whole meal with the appropriate add-ons. When you start filling in with substantial protein like sliced or shredded meats, then you take the salad bar to a whole new level. The number of things you make available is almost infinite. Remember the age of your audience and keep the exotic stuff to a minimum with the younger crowd. To make serving go faster, try combining the basic ingredients (shredded carrots, chopped celery, sliced tomatoes, etc.) in with the lettuce and leave the more exotic toppings on the side.

- Crispy bacon bits
- Chopped olives – black and green
- Blue cheese crumbles
- Shredded cheddar cheese
- Dried fruits (like cranberries)
- Garbanzo beans
- Chopped hard boiled eggs
- Croutons
- Thin slices of meat: flank steak, roasted chicken, barbecue, grilled fish or shrimp

- Sunflower seeds
- Seasoned croutons
- Parmesan cheese
- Pickles (sweet and dill)
- Nuts (sliced almonds, walnuts, pecans)
- Sliced onions or chopped green onions
- Raw veggies (broccoli, cauliflower, cucumber, carrots)
- Crackers

Dressings: Oil and Vinegar, Ranch (light and regular) Blue Cheese, Thousand Island, French
Note: if you are limiting your dressing choices, Oil and Vinegar and Ranch are the most popular.

Hamburger Bar

We all love going to the hamburger place where we get to specify what goes on our burgers. The whole idea of "hold the mayo, heavy on the mustard" is not new. What makes this bar a little different are the sauces you can add to elevate the proceedings. Check out the three sauces in the soups and sandwiches section for some ideas, but hamburgers are like pizza – you can top them with anything that doesn't induce nausea. If you are the one cooking the burgers, try this trick: make an indentation in the middle of the patty with your thumb. This thins out the patty so the center cooks quicker and you don't end up with charred edges and a bloody center. Keep the cooked patties warming in a slow cooker.

- Feta cheese sauce
- Roasted garlic mayonnaise
- Roasted pepper mayonnaise
- Bacon
- Onions, raw or smothered
- Pimento cheese

- Lettuce
- Pickles
- Tomatoes
- Cheeses: cheddar, jack, pepper Jack
- Jalapenos
- Sautéed veggies like onions, peppers and mushrooms, either separate or combined

Condiments: mustard, mayonnaise, ketchup

Waffle Bar

This is a fun bar for a breakfast buffet. Start with prepared frozen waffles. Note: we tried making the waffles fresh one year – disaster! The electric wiring in the room was not set up to accommodate so many waffles irons operating at once. And the delay factor of waiting for a waffle was not pretty. Frozen waffles are pretty darn good and worth their weight in gold for this menu. You could also use frozen French toast.

- Butter
- Whipped cream
- Toasted pecans
- Chocolate chips and sprinkles
- Honey

- Syrup
- Fresh fruit: strawberries, blueberries, bananas, etc.
- Fruit preserves
- Chocolate syrup

If you are planning on serving the ever-popular bacon as an accompaniment to the waffles, consider having a local restaurant cook it for you. They are adept at processing large quantities, and they end up with all that grease rather than you! Check costs – sometimes it isn't that much more expensive than buying the bacon and cooking it yourself. This is a great time-saver and a popular option at pot-lucks for parents who work and don't have the time to cook 20 pounds of bacon.

Sundae Bar

This is possibly one of the most popular food choices for kids of all ages. The ice cream bar is always mobbed at any event. It is a little messy and should be closely supervised if you are using cans of spray topping (it brings out the naughty in children). It is best to have the ice cream already dished out for diners. Be sure you have enough coolers well stocked with ice to keep the ice cream waiting in the wings solid. You might want to limit your ice cream choices to vanilla and chocolate – they make the most popular bases for the toppings. You can use almost anything with sugar in it to top the ice cream. If you have a color theme going (like school colors or a season), you can usually find candy in those colors, especially M&Ms. Any candy you use should not require unwrapping for expediency. Food clubs sell large bottles of flavored syrups. If you need more bottles to spread around the table, decant the syrup from a large container into inexpensive squeeze bottles sold for ketchup or mustard. Add a label.

- Spray whipped cream
- Cookie crumbles
- Candy bar crumbles
- Chocolate chips
- Fresh fruits: bananas, berries, peaches
- Flavored syrups: chocolate, caramel and strawberry
- Nuts: peanuts, pecans, cashews, almonds

- Frozen whipped topping
- Maraschino cherries
- Toasted coconut
- Colored sprinkles

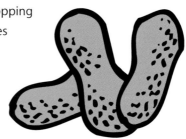

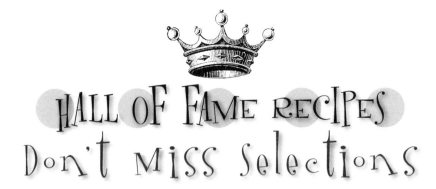

HALL OF FAME RECIPES
Don't Miss Selections

I f you can only try a few recipes from this book, here are some you shouldn't miss. They are some of my most requested recipes:

Nana's Garlic Brisket: tender, succulent, garlicky – this brisket feeds a crowd cheaply and makes your home smell like heaven while it is cooking. It also makes incredible sandwiches with sourdough bread and horseradish sauce. This is my most requested recipe of all time. I keep copies of it on hand whenever I serve it because I have never NOT gotten a request for it after people taste this brisket.

Fried Bread: Unusual and divine, this recipe from my mother is one she ate growing up. Crispy bread dough fried in olive oil is salted or sugared. It is impossible to quit eating this. Kids go nuts for it once they taste it. It is fun to cook when you have a house full of teenagers. Don't plan on going out afterward, though. You will be too full to move comfortably.

Corn Pudding: Shirley Jarvis is a fabulous cook and this is her recipe for using the freshest corn of the season. The corn taste is intense and sweet. It is wrapped in a cloudlike mix of eggs, butter and cream. This is easy to fix and is constantly requested by her adoring family.

Bok Choy Salad: This recipe will surprise you. It is quite addictive. The mix of velvety-smooth bok choy with the sweet/sour/crunchy mix of dressing and topping hits all the right notes. Teenagers really like it.

Mother's Vegetable Soup: This recipe is a family treasure. It is worth the effort of several days slow cooking, although it can be done quickly if need be. The unhurried cooking of broth and meat adds much depth to the flavor. Once all the veggies are added in, you have a nutritious meal in a bowl that can simmer on the stove all winter long.

Spicy Baked Beans: This dish is just one mouthful of intense flavor after another. It is full of sauce, vegetables, even pineapple. It takes baked beans to the next level. You won't want to waste space on the entrée if these beans are on the menu.

Cream Cheese Braids: One of my favorite ways to sin. A sweet dough wraps a cheesecake-like mixture. Soft and rich, it reminds me of eating a Krispy Kreme donut hot out of the oil. This is an amazing Christmas gift to make. Just make sure no one on the gift list has a heart condition…

Cheddar Rosemary Dates: This is such an unusual combination of flavors and textures. Another one of those recipes everyone wants after they taste the dates stuffed with a pecan and covered with a cheddar-rosemary crust. Mmmmm.

Blueberry French Toast: Decadence, thy name is Blueberry French Toast. This dish is creamy, fruity, rich, and actually quite easy to prepare. It makes overnight guests feel indulged. Perfect for the holidays.

MASTERING THE FUNDAMENTALS: In-Depth Recipes

COOKED CHICKEN FOR CASSEROLES

So you have a recipe that calls for cooked, cut up chicken. Where does it come from? A can? If you are in a rush, you could use this option, but a rotisserie chicken from the deli would be a better choice. Even better is a whole chicken you cook yourself – it is easy and tastes the best. Plus you get a nice variety of light and dark meat. Don't let a whole bird intimidate you. You get the most meat for your money with a whole chicken, and you end up with all that wonderful stock you can use in other recipes. All you need is a little extra time and a willingness to get your hands messy. You can use the chicken in casseroles, in a noodle or tortilla soup, chicken and dumplings, on sandwiches, in enchiladas. Freeze what you don't need immediately.

If you want another option, try roasting chicken thighs instead of cooking a whole chicken. There is no long list of ingredients; it's all about the technique. The meat is browned and then roasted; the skin is left on during the cooking process to protect the meat, which remains moist and incredibly flavorful. Leaving the bone in also adds flavor. Like the boiled chicken, roasting the chicken pieces requires a little advance preparation, but you end up with an ingredient that is going to improve any recipe. The roasted thighs are a little less messy to prepare than the boiled chicken, but you don't have the stock when you are finished without an extra step. Try both techniques!

BOILED CHICKEN

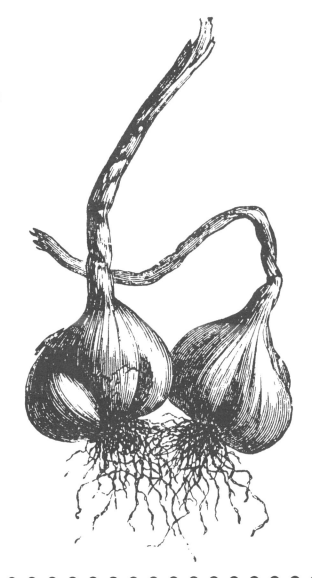

1 whole chicken, either a fryer or roaster, giblets included

Cold water

1 large onion

1-2 ribs celery

3-4 cloves garlic

1-2 carrots

1 bay leaf

Peppercorns

Salt to taste

1. Place the chicken in a deep stock pot and cover completely with cold water.
2. Place over medium high heat and bring to a boil.
3. As the water comes to a boil, skim the scum that floats to the top of the water. All chickens will produce this no matter where they were raised or what they ate. It is a combination of protein from the blood, and melting fat. You will have a cloudy broth if you don't remove it. Once you have removed the scum, add the vegetables, bay leaf, and peppercorns. You don't even need to peel the onion, garlic or carrot, since they will not be eaten; they are simply in there for the flavor. Their skins add a rich color to your broth.
4. Turn the heat down to a simmer and cook the chicken, uncovered, until tender, about an hour. The broth should bubble very, very gently while it cooks; it should not stay at a rolling boil. If the broth cooks way down, don't worry. Just add a little more water (or a splash of wine)?
5. When the chicken is falling from the bones, remove it from the broth to a large platter and spread it out to cool. Don't even try to handle it until it has cooled off.
6. When the meat is comfortable to the touch, peel away all of the skin. Go through and de-bone the chicken – the bones should just pull away from the meat. You will also need to remove the cartilage and skin – anything that isn't meat. You can tear most of the meat into bite-sized pieces with your hands. If you want a more uniform look to your pieces, use the large breast pieces and cut them with a large knife. Lightly salt the meat before storing or using in a recipe.
7. Strain the cooled broth and discard the vegetables. You can lightly salt your broth at this point, if desired. Let the broth cool for an hour before refrigerating it overnight. The fat will float to the top and harden. Remove the fat with a spoon and store or freeze the broth. Remember, if you are freezing the broth in a glass jar, leave about one inch of head room to give the liquid room to expand without breaking the jar. Plastic containers also need the head room for expansion, but they do avoid the bits of broken glass dilemma.

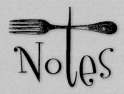

Notes

• *I like to keep two bowls handy while I de-bone the chicken. I put the skin and bones in one bowl (gee, that sounds a little gruesome), and the cleaned meat in the other.*

• *If you are using the chicken in a chicken salad recipe, add a few springs of fresh tarragon to the broth while the chicken cooks. This will lend a wonderful, subtle flavor to the chicken that greatly enhances a mayonnaise concoction.*

• *If you are going to store the chicken for a few days before using it, or if you are going to freeze a portion, add a little broth to the storage container. This will keep the chicken moist and fresh tasting.*

• *Save the fat you skim off the top of the broth and use it for flavoring in a recipe where butter or oil is called for. If you are making the chicken pot pie recipe, be sure to use this chicken fat in your dough. Add in enough of the other fat to the chicken fat to equal the total amount required.*

ROASTED THIGHS

4-5 pounds chicken thighs, skin on
Oil
Salt and pepper

1. Rinse the chicken pieces and pat them dry. This helps them to brown nicely.
2. Sprinkle the pieces with salt and pepper. Cover the bottom of a large skillet with a film of olive oil and heat on medium high. When the oil is hot, add the chicken, cooking it in two batches. Cook the chicken about 10 minutes on each side, until nicely browned. The chicken shouldn't be cooked through and through; this is just a browning step that adds depth of flavor. Remove the pieces to drain on a paper towel. Add more oil to the skillet and repeat with the remaining chicken.
3. Preheat the oven to 350 degrees. Nestle the chicken in a single layer in a large roasting pan. When the oven is heated, add the chicken and roast, uncovered, for an hour. Check during cooking to make sure the meat is not drying out. If it looks like it might be getting dry, make a loose tent over the pan with tinfoil.
4. Remove the chicken from the oven and let it cool about 15 minutes. Put a few pieces of the chicken on a cutting board at a time and remove the skin. Drag the meat from the bone using two forks. Refrigerate meat until ready to use.

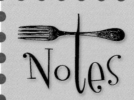

Notes

• You could still get a stock from the thighs – fill the roasting pan halfway with water and place on a large burner. Bring the liquid to a gentle boil and scrape all the tasty bits off the bottom of the pan (this is called de-glazing.) Carefully transfer this water to a large pot and add the thigh bones, skin and juices. Throw in a few cloves of garlic, a piece of onion, a few peppercorns and bring the mixture to a boil. Lower the heat and simmer for about 45 minutes. Cool the broth and strain.

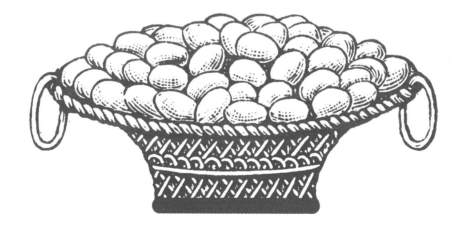

DIVINE DEVILED EGGS

Deviled eggs are like mashed potatoes: they can take on a variety of personalities, depending on the additions to the basic recipe. But nothing beats the humble boiled egg mashed with a few unsurprising ingredients. A survey of recipes reveals that mustard and mayonnaise are the primary - and most important - additions to boiled eggs for traditional deviled eggs. These two ingredients give deviled eggs their familiar, comfort-food taste. In fact, when I have just one boiled egg rolling around the refrigerator, I simply cut it in half, slather on a little mayonnaise and dribble just a bit of mustard over each half, add a sprinkle of salt and let my mouth do all the blending. It is a fast and neat way to enjoy a devilish egg without the bowls and mashing.

I prefer using a full-fat mayonnaise for deviled eggs because the mashed filling has much more body than one made with low-fat mayonnaise. Some recipes call for a large quantity of mayonnaise – as much as $1/2$ cup per 6-8 eggs. I would rather use a little

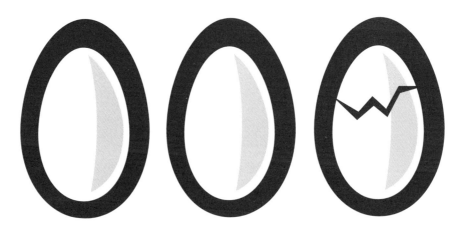

less mayonnaise, but stick with the full-fat variety. I find about ¹/₄ cup is plenty to moisten 6-8 eggs. If you are trying to cut down on fat and calories, add the mayonnaise in stages until you reach your desired consistency. Start with a scant tablespoon.

Mustard is a wild card. It can be simple and somewhat anonymous, or you can indulge in a lovely, grainy variety, or one with added flavor, like horseradish or wasabi. Don't be afraid to experiment with something other than plain yellow mustard in your eggs. Dijon is my favorite addition. It adds an interesting level of flavor without commanding too much attention.

After playing with a lot of deviled egg recipes, I discovered the secret ingredient for the best deviled eggs is a squirt of fresh lemon juice. I know it sounds a little strange, but the lemon juice brightens and intensifies flavors that otherwise might be bland or mushy. You don't taste the lemon at all, just its beneficial effect.

Other traditional ingredients include onion, celery and relish. Since one of the appeals of deviled eggs is the contrasting textures of the firm whites and the smooth filling, it is important that these ingredients be minced finely to preserve the filling's smoothness. Any or all of these ingredients can be added to your basic mash of yolk, mayonnaise and mustard. A little sprinkle of salt and a dash of either white pepper or hot sauce, and you have comfort food of the highest order. I like to add some minced parsley as well, for the color and for the fresh taste it brings. A garnish of paprika for some lovely color and you are done.

I think it is important to taste as you go when you make deviled eggs. I always seem to have an odd number of eggs and end up guesstimating quantities. Use the recipe below as a blueprint, a starting point for modification. An extra egg or two shouldn't affect your quantities much. If you like your eggs a little moister, you will need to add a bit more mayonnaise or mustard. If your onion smells really strong while you mince it, you might want to use only half and taste before adding more. If you are adding additional spices, tasting is critical.

Deviled eggs lend themselves beautifully to variations. If you want a spicy Mexican egg, substitute fresh cilantro for the parsley and add a sprinkle (or two) of chipotle chili powder. You could even use a spicy mustard. And you can always add chopped jalapeno as a little surprise for the palate.

An Italian egg might have some fresh oregano chopped up with the parsley. A sprinkle of Italian salad dressing base and the tiniest drizzle of olive oil added to the mashed yolks ups the flavor. Finish with a shaving of Parmesan cheese.

Try an Asian egg using wasabi mustard, a tiny little squirt of sesame oil to supplement a bare minimum of mayonnaise, and finish with a sprinkle of toasted sesame seeds.

I have made deviled eggs using ranch dressing, and they were a big hit with a lot of people. Try it (or another creamy salad dressing from a bottle) sometime when you are in a hurry or bored with the usual renditions. Finish with a hearty sprinkle of crispy bacon.

Cooking an egg for mashing is simple, but it requires attention. High heat is not an egg's friend, whether scrambling or boiling. It toughens the egg. Instead of boiling the life out of an egg for 20 minutes try this method instead.

• To boil eggs: put the eggs right from the refrigerator into a pot and cover them with cold water. Heat the water over a medium high heat; when the water comes to a boil, lower the heat and cover. Simmer the eggs over low heat (the water should just barely break with bubbles) for 8 minutes, then remove from the heat and let them sit, covered, for another ten minutes. Drain and cover with cold water to cool before peeling.

• To peel eggs: crack them gently on the counter in 4-5 different spots, and then roll them in your hands, applying gentle pressure. Return to the bowl of water and peel the eggs while they are submerged. This helps dislodge any clinging shell. When you crack an egg on a sharp edge, it can drive the shell up into the egg. Rolling is better.

Try baking eggs instead of boiling for egg salad or deviled eggs. You can cook a large number easily this way. Baking eggs gives them a lovely creamy texture.

• To bake eggs: place one oven rack in the center of the oven. Position the second rack one or two levels below. Place a baking sheet on the bottom rack to catch any eggs that might break. Preheat the oven to 325 degrees. Place the eggs on the top rack and bake for 30 minutes. Remove and immediately place in a cold-water bath to stop the cooking and cool for easy handling.

Don't be alarmed at any brown spots you see on baked eggs. Some of the egg white seeps out of the shell during baking and it caramelizes in the heat. While interesting to look at, this occurrence doesn't affect texture, taste, or volume.

• **Another preparation tip:** for easy clean-up, put all the hard-cooked yolks in a large zip-top bag and seal. Mash yolks with your hand or a rolling pin until broken up. Add the remaining ingredients, squishing around in the bag until they are all mixed. Snip off a small bit of the bag at the corner and squirt the filling through the small hole into the egg whites. Just throw away the bag when you are done. I would use this method only if you aren't experimenting with ingredients and don't need to taste.

This zip-bag trick is a great way to transport deviled eggs without angst. Leave the prepared yolks in the bag and toss all the empty whites in another zip-top bag. When you get to your destination, snip a corner of the bag and fill the egg whites.

BASIC DEVILED EGGS ●

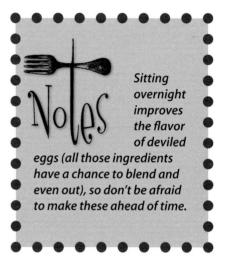

8 eggs, hard-cooked and peeled (see instructions for cooking above)

$^1/_4$ cup high quality, full-fat mayonnaise (I prefer Hellmann's)

Juice from half a fresh lemon

1 tablespoon full-flavored mustard

2 tablespoons finely minced celery (optional)

1 tablespoon finely minced onion, either green or sweet white onion (optional)

1-2 tablespoons pickle relish (optional)

1-2 tablespoons finely chopped fresh parsley, either curly or flat-leaf

$^1/_2$ - 1 teaspoon salt, or to taste

Several dashes hot sauce

Paprika for garnish

Notes

Sitting overnight improves the flavor of deviled eggs (all those ingredients have a chance to blend and even out), so don't be afraid to make these ahead of time.

1. Slice cooked eggs in half and separate the white from the yolks. Put the yolks in a small mixing bowl and mash with the back of a fork until they resemble very fine-grained cornmeal.
2. Squeeze the lemon over the yolks and stir in the mayonnaise and mustard and any remaining ingredients you are using – celery, onion, relish, parsley, salt and pepper or hot sauce. Mix gently until the mixture forms a nice, smooth paste. Taste and correct seasonings, adding more mayonnaise to reach the desired consistency.
3. Fill the whites with the yolk paste, mounding up generously. Garnish with a sprinkle of paprika. Refrigerate until ready to use.

ODE TO MASHED POTATOES

I n this low-carb world, mashed potatoes are the best way to sin. Their warm, creamy richness makes them the ultimate comfort food and perfect foil for any animal protein offering.

There are as many variations for mashed potatoes as there are recipes for chili. Some involve using chicken broth instead of cream to save calories (only if you MUST – mashed potatoes are about indulgence, not good sense). "Dirty" potatoes have the skin left on for more texture and nutrition. And then, there are those fabulous add-ins. The unassuming personality of potatoes makes them the perfect vehicle for brighter, stronger flavors. Check out combinations like rosemary and roasted garlic, blue cheese and caramelized onions, smoked cheddar and grainy mustard – the possibilities are endless.

But let's start with plain, unadorned mashed potatoes. The procedure is quite simple: boil, mash, season. (Note: I have never used a recipe to make mashed potatoes. I just add things to the potatoes gradually until I like their consistency; amounts differ according to which ingredients you choose.)

The first step is to boil the potatoes. Water temperature is an important player here. You should put the potatoes in cold salted water and heat them together, rather than dropping the potatoes into already boiling water as you typically do when boiling vegetables. When food hits water that is already boiling, more of the flavor and vitamins remain in it.

With potatoes, another factor is at play: mushiness. If you drop potatoes into boiling water, the outside cooks quicker than the inside; the outside is mushy by the time the inside is cooked. Starting the potatoes in cold water evens out their texture since the slow heating allows the inside to cook before the outside texture goes south.

Another consideration is what to do to the potato before it goes in the water. Just peel it and cut it into large chunks, right? Well, maybe. Some recipes recommend leaving the skin on potatoes while they boil to prevent them from absorbing so much cooking water. The resulting drier potatoes absorb more flavor when they are seasoned. Cooled in a bowl of cold water, they can be peeled with your hands.

Some recipes go a step further: the potato is boiled unpeeled and uncut. This ultimate flavor-saver technique of boiling the potato whole takes considerably more time than cooking potato chunks. Which way is best? I have prepared potatoes all three ways, and to tell the truth, I can't tell much difference. I like to boil them in large, unpeeled chunks.

Another pre-cooking option is to rinse the cut potatoes in several changes of water. This removes excess starch and keeps the potatoes from getting gummy when you mash them. It adds one more step to simple mashed potatoes, but it is worth the effort.

Whichever way you decide to cook the potatoes, how do you know when they are done? To test for doneness, pull a potato chunk from the water and insert a knife into it. Wiggle the knife a little bit. The potato should fall apart. If it doesn't split, boil it a little longer. If it disintegrates, oops – it cooked too long.

Once your potatoes are properly cooked, drain them and return them to the pot. Place the pot back on the burner to dry out any lingering moisture (and watch carefully that they don't burn).

Now you are ready to mash. Mashing can be done with a potato ricer, which produces the smoothest results, but is a little tedious and messy. You place a cooked potato in the ricer and press the potato through the small holes. The result is small, rice-shaped pieces of potato (hence the name). A good old-fashioned hand masher works well, too, especially if you like leaving some "homemade" lumps in the mixture. You can use an electric mixer, but be careful – you can quickly overwork the potatoes, which produces a gummy mess.

Seasonings can be added before you mash the potatoes so they are well-incorporated. I always start with a good dose of salt and pepper. You will need quite a bit of salt to bring up the flavor of the potatoes, since they are pretty bland without it. Start small and add gradually. I find it takes quite a few tastes to get the amount right. (Darn!) When you are ready to add a little heat, use white pepper. It imparts a distinctive flavor and mellow heat without a bite. Just as important, it doesn't scar the lovely white potato surface with unsightly black dots.

If you are adding butter (and who doesn't?), add it next. Unsalted butter, with its sweet, fresh taste, is my first choice. To me, it is the most important flavoring ingredient in mashed potatoes, and I gauge the amount of liquid to be added only after the butter has been incorporated. If you add the butter last, you might end up with a too-thin mixture – or worse, one that isn't buttery enough because you didn't want to thin down the consistency.

Next, slowly add a warmed liquid: heavy cream, half and half, regular or skim milk, or sour cream. Add enough liquid to produce a fluffy but not too-thin concoction; the potatoes should mound and hold their shape, rather than run off the spoon like thick icing. The amounts of liquid you will need to produce this result will vary depending on the viscosity of the liquid you use. You will need more of the heavier/thicker liquids. Try using a combination of liquids - something I did out of necessity once due to a cream shortage, and found I preferred it! I use our regular skim or 2 percent milk for most of the liquid, and then throw in a bit of sour cream for texture and tartness. Gently warm your liquids before you add them to your potatoes to keep everything nice and hot.

Taste one more time for salt and pepper. Finish with a generous pat of butter melted into the middle of your potato mound and you are ready for a little bit of heaven.

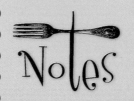

Notes

• White potatoes, with their higher starch content, produce a lighter, fluffier texture but they tend to be on the bland side. Russet potatoes have an earthy potato flavor, and their high starch content enables them to bind beautifully with cream and butter. Yukon Golds have a creamy, buttery texture with sweet golden overtones. Either Russets or Golds make a grand mash.

• Make potatoes ahead and keep them warm in a slow cooker. Adjust their consistency with cream before serving.

• When holding prepared potatoes on the stove top, place a dish towel between the lid and pot to absorb excess moisture from condensation.

• Sometimes you might want to make the potatoes ahead. Do the cooking early and hold cooked potatoes, either riced or in chunks, in a zip top bag. When you are ready to serve, heat them in the microwave and then mash, adding warmed cream and seasoning at the last minute.

• Red potatoes hold their shape for potato salad better than white or Russet potatoes. Their thin skin makes them a good choice for "dirty" mashed potatoes, too.

• If you are adding garlic to your potatoes, roast it first and add the paste. Or simmer peeled, sliced, or mashed garlic in the butter you will add later on. Bring the garlic and butter to a boil, then lower the heat and let them simmer for about 15 minutes (longer is OK). Remove the garlic before incorporating the butter. Using this garlic-flavored butter instead of raw garlic imparts a more subtle flavor – one that won't give you nightmares.

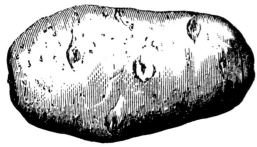

MUSINGS ON MEATLOAF

Meatloaf is humble. It doesn't aspire to be anything but what it is: ground meat all flavored up and baked in a loaf. It is the perfect foundation for mashed potatoes. It also can be part of a spectacular sandwich. It is one of those ultimate comfort foods that gets overlooked because it is mostly brown and cheap. But simple doesn't mean boring. Let's take a look at the key ingredients in a meatloaf and consider the possibilities. Here are some tips to make your meatloaf an exciting dish your family and friends will request again and again.

Meat: Not surprisingly, meatloaf benefits from the right kind of meat. Ground chuck, at 80 percent lean, is terrific for hamburgers cooked on the grill, where all that fat drips away, perhaps starting a small fire. With a meatloaf, you'll miss that kind of excitement. You want something less fatty, since the meat will be sitting in its juices during the cooking process. (But it doesn't have to – more on that later.) Ground sirloin, high in flavor and lower in fat, is a good starting point. But you don't want to use only sirloin, because you will have one dry baby of a loaf. Half chuck and half sirloin is a safe, tasty combination. But consider combining more than one meat in your loaf. You will need a total of about 2- 2 $^1/_2$ pounds for a nice, family-sized loaf. A half pound of sirloin and a half pound chuck is a good beginning. The other meats you add are for flavor and texture. Ground veal is a fancy addition that improves both without adding a distinctive flavor of its own. I also like to use bulk pork sausage or ground pork for their flavor. Breakfast sausage adds lots of flavor and even a little heat if you select the spicy variety. You could use a pound of mixed ground beef and a pound of sausage. Or try around $^1/_2$ pound each of ground veal and pork/pork sausage added to a pound of sirloin/chuck mix. See? Isn't this fun?

Breadcrumbs: Sure, you can use the stuff that comes in a can, but those prepared crumbs make your meatloaf tough, according to Martha Stewart's crack team of chefs. They prefer homemade bread crumbs (of course!) made by pulsing white bread in a food processor. This idea is good as far as it goes. Why not use other bread options: sourdough, whole wheat, or a firm-textured bread like an Italian loaf or a boule that creates a little texture without adding too much flavor? Another great option is to use salad croutons, pre-seasoned and crunchy. Buzz up about 6 ounces in a processor and add to your meatloaf. You can choose from a huge variety of crouton flavors.

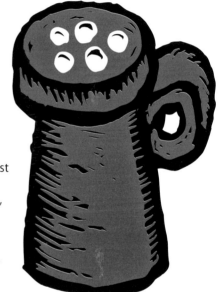

Vegetables: Yes? No? Maybe so? Most recipes add a little something from the plant world, most often onions, carrots, celery, and green peppers. And garlic – at least one clove and usually 2-3 (when you combine garlic with meat, more is more. I always opt for 3 promising-looking cloves, nice and fat and unsprouted.) The vegetables' watery nature adds moisture to the loaf, and of course, they have nice health implications. But they need to be cut up quite small to ensure even cooking and anonymity within the whole. You don't want any ingredient interrupting the smoothness and homogenous flavor of a good meatloaf. Pulse the veggies in a food processor until they are quite small but not pureed.

Seasonings: In addition to the de rigueur salt and pepper, you have a choice of fresh or dried herbs like rosemary or thyme, which is particularly good with meat. If you are doing an Italian-slant loaf, you might want a little oregano and basil, too. I always like a little fresh parsley, flat or curly – about $^1/_2$ cup. For fun, you can add spices too, for bits of zing: cumin, chili powder, chipotle powder. Just shake a little over your bowl (or to be more precise, try about $^1/_2$ - 1 teaspoon). Each time I make meatloaf, I use something a little different, depending on my mood and what the herb garden is doing.

Ketchup: this iconic sauce has to show up somewhere in your loaf - either mixed in with the meat, used in a glaze on top, or puddled on the plate for dipping. I like mine on top. My favorite glaze fuses ketchup with sweet brown sugar or honey, and savory mustard. It turns into a thick, sticky sauce as it bakes into the loaf, delivering a punch of sweet/savory flavor with each bite.

Loafiness: we used to cook our loaves in a "meatloaf pan", and the poor little meat mound boiled in its own juices during cooking. No more; evolution is a beautiful thing. Now you can shape your meat (but carefully – too much rough handling will make it heavy and dense) and bake it on a cookie sheet. This method gives the loaf a nice crust all the way around and enables fats and excess moisture to drain away. You can either bake the shaped loaf directly on the cookie sheet, or, for even more drainage, you can suspend the meat on a cooling rack placed on a cookie sheet lined with parchment paper or aluminum foil to catch the drippings. Sounds crazy, but it works; it is my preferred cooking method.

Lagniappe: One of my favorite meatloaf recipes uses thinly sliced onions sautéed in a little olive oil and scattered over the glaze on top of the loaf before cooking. They crisp up in the oven and take on the character of a fried onion ring without the guilt of batter and extra oil. Try it!!

FAVORITE MEATLOAF RECIPE ●

This recipe has evolved over the years, borrowing from many different sources and always is a work in progress. It uses a wonderful variety of meat and flavored croutons, and then finishes with crispy onion rings on a spicy sweet topping.

6 ounces seasoned croutons

$^1/_2$ teaspoon cayenne pepper

1 teaspoon dried thyme

1 teaspoon chili powder (chipotle preferred)

1 teaspoon cumin

3 cloves of garlic

1 rib celery

1 large carrot, peeled

$^1/_2$ - 1 whole onion (about 1 cup)

$^1/_2$ green or red bell pepper, seeded

1 pound ground sirloin or $^1/_2$ pound each ground sirloin and chuck

1 pound pork breakfast sausage, mild or hot

$^1/_2$ pound ground veal

2 teaspoons salt

2 eggs, beaten

$^1/_2$ cup chopped parsley

Dash of hot sauce (optional)

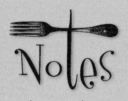

TOPPING

$^1/_2$ cup ketchup

2 tablespoons brown sugar

1 tablespoon spicy brown mustard

1 sweet onion, sliced into very thin rings

1 tablespoon olive oil

1. Preheat the oven to 400 degrees. Line a cookie sheet with parchment paper or aluminum foil. Spray a cooling rack with non-stick spray and place the cooling rack on the covered cookie sheet. Set aside.

2. In a food processor, combine the croutons, cayenne pepper, thyme, chili powder and cumin and buzz until pulverized. Pour into a bowl and set the mixture aside.

3. Put the garlic in the bowl of the processor and pulse until finely chopped. Add the onion, celery, carrot, and bell pepper. Pulse carefully until the vegetables are in fine pieces. Be careful not to over-process; you don't want a puree, just finely chopped vegetables. Turn into a large mixing bowl.

4. To the vegetables add the sirloin, sausage, veal, salt, beaten eggs, parsley and crouton mixture. Combine carefully with your hands. Resist the impulse to squeeze.

5. Gently pat the mixture into a loaf shape (it will be quite large) and place on the cooling rack/prepared cookie sheet.

6. Combine the ketchup, brown sugar and mustard in a small bowl and mix well. Spread evenly over the top of the loaf.

7. Heat the oil in a skillet. When it is hot, add the onions and cook over medium heat. If the onions start to stick or dry out, add a little water and continue cooking until the moisture is evaporated and the onions are soft and a lovely golden color. Spread the onions on top of the loaf over the ketchup mixture.

8. Bake the loaf at 400 degrees for 45 minutes, then turn the oven down to 350 and continue baking another 30 minutes, or until a thermometer inserted into the center reads 160 degrees. Let the loaf sit for 15 minutes before slicing and serving.

Serves 8-10

Notes

• *I like to start the onions for the topping cooking early in the loaf assembly process so they can cook long and slow. They don't take a lot of monitoring. Then they are ready to go when you get your meatloaf shaped.*

• *Depending on how thick you shape your loaf, you may need to cook the loaf longer than 75 minutes. This is where a thermometer is indispensable. If you want a shorter cooking time, shape meat into two smaller loaves. If you do two loaves, you may want to cook up a little more onion and throw together a little extra topping since you will have more surface area to cover. Just add an extra squeeze of ketchup, use heaping spoons of mustard and sugar. It is not an exact science. But it is yummy!*

• *Try using spiced ketchup in the topping. I love the one that has jalapenos in it.*

• *This quantity of chili powder gives a robust flavor without heat. However, if you are a real chile-phobe cut the amount to $^1/_2$ teaspoon or eliminate.*

• *If you don't have croutons, you can use 1 cup breadcrumbs, either packaged or homemade. And if you only have one egg, don't worry. Just add the breadcrumbs slowly so you don't get too dry a texture.*

PerFect Pasta

Pasta is perfect crowd food – it is easy to prepare in quantities, it is inexpensive, filling, and capable of taking on a variety of personalities. A few easy-to-follow guidelines will make cooking this favorite failure-proof.

The pot: You will need a large one - at least a 6-quart (24 cups) capacity - to guard against boil-overs. Handles will make draining the pasta easier.

Water: Have you ever had a sticky mass of noodles when you cooked your pasta? It is because you didn't use enough water. Pasta leeches starch as it cooks, and you want to have plenty of water to dilute the starch and keep it from sticking to the noodles. You need 4 quarts of water to cook 1 pound of pasta. Be sure to stir the pasta as soon as it hits the water to keep it from sticking to the bottom of the pot and massing together in a giant wad. Frequent stirring while it cooks helps as well. Also, do NOT rinse the pasta after you drain it, even though you have seen recipe after recipe tell you to do this. If you used enough cooking water, your noodles won't be sticky because the water diluted all the starch that makes for sticky noodles. Rinsing the noodles will wash away the residual starch that helps the sauce to stick.

Salt: don't be shy. Your one chance to really season the pasta itself (rather than have salt just sitting on top of the cooked pasta) is with the cooking water. It takes more salt than you think to properly season pasta. Use 1 tablespoon of regular salt or 2 tablespoons kosher salt (which has less sodium and tastes less salty) per 4 quarts water/1 pound pasta.

Oil: Don't. Never add oil to the cooking water. It won't keep the noodles from sticking together (only enough cooking water will do that), and it will make the noodles slippery and prevent a sauce from adhering. Big disappointment. I don't care what your mama told you, just don't do it. Now, adding oil to the noodles after they are cooked and have been drained is a completely different proposition. Go for it! Pasta tossed with a little high quality olive oil, a sprinkle of fresh Parmesan cheese and a grate of black pepper is an exquisite simple dinner.

Pasta: figure on one pound of dried pasta to feed four to six people. The number of servings varies depending on whether the pasta is a main dish (4 servings) or side dish (6 servings); whether the sauce is a light tomato sauce (4) or rich Alfredo (6); or whether there are other ingredients like vegetables, meat or seafood, that bulk up each serving.

Al Dente: This is the degree to which pasta is perfectly cooked. Al dente ("to the tooth") means your pasta has a little bite, or stiffness, left in it. Mushy noodles still taste pretty good (so if you overcook yours, for heaven's sake, don't throw them out!), but they lose that nice texture that is such an important part of a well-prepared dish. The best place to start for an idea of how long to cook the pasta is the back of the box in which it came. Subtract 3-4 minutes from the recommended time and start testing the pasta at that point. Remember that the pasta will continue to cook for about 30 seconds while it is draining. Forget throwing the pasta against the wall to see if it sticks. Instead, bite into a piece of pasta to test for doneness. You should be able to see a very faint, whitish center. Or just taste the darn thing and note if it has a little resistance left. Done! If you are using fresh pasta, stay on your toes. It cooks much more quickly than dried pasta since it doesn't need to soften and absorb moisture.

Warming: pasta cools quite quickly, so warm the serving bowl before serving. A neat trick is to place the serving bowl under the colander when you drain the pasta. The hot water will quickly heat your serving bowl and it will be ready and waiting for your pasta. Another option is to place the empty bowl in the microwave and heat for a minute. Check after 30 seconds and continue in 30 second increments so you don't overheat your bowl.

Reserved cooking water: Always save about a cup of the pasta cooking water for use in your sauce. This is the experienced Italian cook's secret ingredient. Some sauce recipes actually call for the pasta water as an ingredient. It is full of starch, so it will help your sauce really cling to the noodles. Use the pasta water to thin a sauce down.

WELL-COOKED PASTA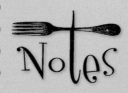

To feed 4-6 you will need to:

1. Place 4 quarts (16 cups) of water and 2 tablespoons kosher salt (or 1 tablespoon regular table salt) in a 6-quart pot. Bring water to a rolling boil. The water should be moving vigorously before you add the pasta.
2. Drop pasta into boiling water, stirring as soon as the pasta hits the water.
3. Turn the heat down to medium high once the water returns to a boil. It should not simmer, however; the water needs to continue to move vigorously. Stir the pasta frequently. Cook pasta until al dente; time will vary according to the pasta you are using. Check the back of the pasta package, then subtract 3-4 minutes from the recommended cooking time and start testing.
5. When the pasta is al dente, ladle $1/2$ - 1 cup of the cooking water into a measuring cup and reserve.
6. Place the colander over the serving bowl and drain pasta, allowing the hot water to sit in the serving bowl for a moment. Do not rinse the pasta.
7. Pour the water out of the serving bowl and fill with cooked pasta. Toss the pasta with a few tablespoons of high quality olive oil and then spoon on the sauce, if using. Toss noodles to distribute the sauce evenly. Finish with a grind of black pepper.

Notes

• *It is especially important that you toss the sauce with the noodles if you are serving the dish on a buffet. You want to make sure the sauce is evenly distributed and all the noodles are coated. Nothing is worse than being the last person in line when you get to the pasta bowl and all that is left is sticky noodles (why wasn't there a little olive oil in there? Or didn't you use enough water when you boiled the pasta?) and no sauce. Besides – a puddle of sauce on top of a mound of noodles is the American version of spaghetti. Italians mix the sauce in well before serving.*

• *My favorite brand of pasta ever? Makaira Pasta alla Chitarra, available from A.G. Ferrari Foods (see ingredients chapter). It is organic, rough-textured (so a sauce really clings), and so full of flavor you can't believe it shares a heritage with the pasta on the grocery store shelf. Pricey, and worth every penny for a splurge meal.*

ROASTED VEGETABLES

This is one fabulous way to prepare veggies – roasting them in the oven with high heat intensifies their flavor and none of their vitamins are leached out into cooking water. You can crisp up some veggies, like potato chips, without the added fat from frying. It is an easy way to prepare large quantities of food in a calorie-conscious way. This method works for almost any vegetable, and it is satisfyingly easy to vary the flavors. You'll get hooked on this recipe and start roasting everything in the fridge!

Desired quantity of vegetables (choose one or a mixture):

> **Asparagus, tough ends removed**
>
> **Eggplant peeled and sliced or diced**
>
> **Potatoes, sweet or white, peeled or unpeeled, cubed, sliced or cut in strips**
>
> **Carrots, peeled and sliced (unpeeled if using baby carrots)**
>
> **Onions, peeled and quartered or sliced**
>
> **Summer squash, sliced**
>
> **Winter squash, unpeeled and split in half**
>
> **Mushrooms, wiped cleaned and sliced or left whole**
>
> **Peppers, sliced in strips**
>
> **Okra, cap removed then sliced**

Seasonings:
Fine quality olive oil
Seasoned salt and fresh-ground black pepper
Fresh garlic, minced (optional)
Fresh herbs and spices (optional)
Balsamic vinegar (optional)
Freshly grated Parmesan cheese (optional)

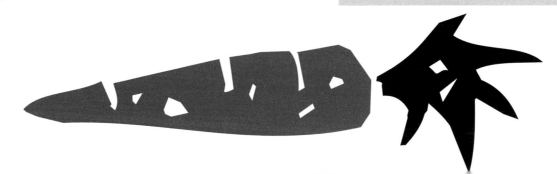

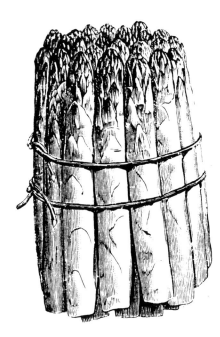

1. Preheat the oven to 400 degrees. Prepare a shallow cookie sheet by lining it with tinfoil or parchment paper. You don't need to oil the pan since the veggies have oil on them.
2. In a large bowl, toss the prepared vegetables with olive oil. The vegetables should be well-coated, but the oil should not pool once the vegetables are on the baking sheet.
3. Season the vegetables with salt and pepper. If you are using garlic, add it now. Mix thoroughly with your hands.
4. Spread the vegetable out on the cookie sheet in a single layer. Use more than one sheet, if necessary to keep them from piling up on each other. If they are more than a single layer deep, they will steam instead of roast, and the flavor won't be as intense.
5. Roast for 30-45 minutes, depending on your vegetable. For example, mushrooms will cook faster than winter squash, so start checking after 30 minutes.
6. Serve hot or room-temperature, finished with a splash of vinegar or sprinkle of Parmesan cheese if desired.

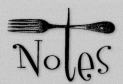

Notes

- *Your choice of seasonings is limitless. You can use a no-salt blend, or one of the many spicy-hot Cajun blends. Try a variety to find your favorite. Or vary them according to the veggie you use.*
- *Add fresh herbs for a big flavor punch. Rosemary and chives work beautifully with potatoes, especially sweet potatoes. A mix of rosemary, oregano and basil are great with eggplant and tomatoes. Tarragon is nice with lighter vegetables like summer squash. Or sprinkle some cinnamon on winter squash. But don't feel pressured to figure out which herb or spice to use if you aren't experimental; the veggies are wonderful plainly roasted with just a little salt, pepper and oil.*
- *When fixing asparagus, I like to use the skinny baby asparagus –it gets crunchy like chips. Even the kids love them. If you want to be fancy, use only the tenderest upper part of the asparagus stalk.*
- *Mix it up! Try eggplant, onions, tomatoes and mushrooms together; peppers and onions (great on hot roast beef or chicken sandwiches); a mix of zucchini and yellow squash; onions and potatoes with big flakes of black pepper – the possibilities are endless. If you are using a number of different vegetables in one batch, try to cut them so all the pieces are the same size. This ensures they will cook evenly.*
- *Roast a big batch of veggies at the beginning of the week, then use them throughout the week tucked inside an omelet for breakfast sprinkled with fresh Parmesan; on a homemade pizza; tossed with some pasta; baked inside puff pastry. Throw them in a soup or tomato sauce for deep flavor; puree them first for a smooth soup.*
- *This is a wonderful alternative to fried veggies, particularly okra, which gets crisp instead of slimy.*

SALAD DRESSING BASICS

No longer a wallflower at the buffet table, salads have become an essential part of most meals. They please the vegetarians, the weight-conscious, and the health-conscious. They can be composed with extravagant ingredients or remain spartan. No matter what you put in the salad, though, what goes on the salad can make or break the dish.

As I have noted numerous times, bottled Ranch dressing is the hands-down favorite of most kids, and it makes a tempting dip for raw veggies. Well, maybe not tempting, but kids will dip just about anything in it for flavor camouflage.

The most versatile dressing, and my personal favorite, is the vinaigrette, a divine duo of oil and vinegar. You can use these two simple ingredients to dress lettuce, roasted veggies, potato salad, even fruit salad. Use it as a marinade for grilled meats. It makes almost anything taste better. Flavorful additions to this simple base recipe are endless.

The ratio of oil to vinegar varies from recipe to recipe, with some recipes using 4 parts oil to one part vinegar – a very traditional take on vinaigrette – while other, more calorie/health conscious recipes use a 3:1 ratio, which has less oil and a more prominent vinegar flavor. It really depends on your taste buds and your ingredients. A stouter, more strongly-flavored vinegar like balsamic can be used more sparingly than soft vinegars, like rice or champagne vinegar. If the vinegar is light-colored, it is usually milder than a dark vinegar. Use the 4:1 combination with dark vinegars and the 3:1 ratio with light, mild vinegars.

If you really want a flavor boost, try reducing balsamic vinegar in a small pan on the stovetop over low heat for about 10-15 minutes. The flavors become really concentrated. Doing this with an inexpensive, grocery store balsamic vinegar will bring it closer to the flavor of an expensive aged balsamic. Use the reduced vinegar in combination with oil for a dressing or splash on fresh fruit for a wonderfully refreshing dessert.

You can also use other acidic liquids in a salad dressing instead of, or in combination with, vinegar, like fresh lemon or lime juice. You get about 2 tablespoons of juice per lemon or lime. The citrus brightens the flavor of a salad and allows the personality of your greens or vegetables to really shine through. Treat these liquids like a light vinegar and use the 3:1 combination. Or try using half vinegar, half citrus juice in a recipe. This will add layers of flavor.

With such a simple concoction, the quality of your ingredients becomes critical. Use a good quality olive oil, although you needn't spend the really big bucks on olive oil for salad dressing since its flavor will be somewhat masked by the additional ingredients. While a great oil is unnecessary, a crummy one will absolutely degrade the flavor of your finished dish. Stick with a mid-priced oil that has a lovely, fruity aroma. If you happen to have a really high quality (i.e. expensive!) olive oil, try using it alone, drizzled at the last minute over your salad and finished with a grind of black pepper. This is a wonderful finish for really fresh baby lettuces or salads that combine strong, interesting flavors like cranberries, Feta and walnuts.

Olive oil has all kinds of health benefits, but canola oil is a good choice for dressing, too. It has a milder flavor than olive oil, so vinegar flavors will be more pronounced. Use the 4:1 ratio with canola oil unless you are interested in ramping up the tartness of the dressing.

Once you have your basic oil/vinegar measured out, you can start adding flavors. Always, you will want some salt and fresh-ground pepper. A good rule of thumb is a teaspoon of salt per cup of oil. Use half that amount (1/2 teaspoon) of pepper.

Another good addition to almost any vinaigrette dressing is a pinch of mustard. I prefer prepared mustard, although some recipes use dry mustard. Prepared mustard comes in a wonderful variety of flavors, not just yellow and Dijon. The creamy texture mixes easily with the oil and vinegar. Try an exotic blend, like jalapeno or chipotle mustard, for a change of pace. Start with about $^1/_2$ - 1 teaspoon of mustard per cup of oil, and add more as desired.

If you want to add garlic to your dressing without the nightmares that raw garlic can produce, you have several options. Mash a clove of garlic with the side of a wide knife and place the crushed clove in the olive oil you are using for the salad. Let it marinate in the oil for a few hours, and then remove it before adding the rest of the ingredients to the oil.

Or, take a page from Caesar salad prep and rub a wooden salad bowl with a mashed piece of garlic until the bowl is coated with the juice. Toss out the garlic and add the vinaigrette, rolling it around the bowl to pick up the garlic flavoring.

Another option is to use roasted garlic instead of raw garlic. It gives a mellow, rich flavor to the dressing that combines well with blue cheese or bacon bits. To roast garlic, take an entire head of garlic (made up of multiple cloves) and cut off just a bit of the pointed end so the interior is exposed. Place the garlic in a double layer of tinfoil folded up to make a pouch. Drizzle garlic with olive oil, sprinkle with salt, and seal. Roast in a 350-degree oven for 35-40 minutes. Remove and cool. Squeeze the garlic paste out of each clove into a dish. Use a fork to blend and even out the texture. Add the paste to the olive oil for your vinaigrette and blend well before combing with other ingredients.

An alternative to fresh or roasted garlic is garlic powder. It won't have the same vibrancy of flavor, but it will add a wonderful note of its own. Use about $^1/_2$ teaspoon per cup of oil. Ditto onion powder.

A trick I learned from my mother-in-law when making salad with vinaigrette dressing is to put your mixed dressing in the bottom of the salad bowl first. (This makes it easy to eyeball your proportions of oil and vinegar.) Add your veggies like cucumbers, carrots, tomatoes, onions, peppers, etc. and let them marinate in the dressing while you finish the salad. Pile on the lettuce last of all, and then toss with the marinated vegetables. Top with finishers like bacon, sunflower seeds, and croutons.

Rule of thumb for estimating how much salad and dressing you need: allow 1 cup of greens per person and 1-2 tablespoons of dressing per serving. If you are using a creamy dressing, you will need more since it doesn't slip over the greens as easily to coat them. Add dressing a little at a time to avoid an irredeemably soggy salad. Keep dressing in the refrigerator for up to three weeks. Allow to warm up to room temperature before adding to greens.

BASIC VINAIGRETTE (MILD) ●

For the vinaigrette:

$^1/_4$ **cup vinegar, or $^1/_2$ and $^1/_2$ mix of vinegar and lemon or lime juice**

1 cup nice quality olive oil

1 teaspoon salt or to taste

$^1/_2$ **teaspoon freshly ground black pepper**

Add-ins:

1 teaspoon Dijon mustard

1 clove garlic, finely minced (see notes for other ways to add garlic flavor)

1 tablespoon fresh, chopped herbs: basil, chives, oregano, rosemary, tarragon, thyme, cilantro, mint, dill, parsley (see notes)

1 tablespoon minced red or green onion

$^1/_2$ **teaspoon garlic powder (instead of the fresh garlic)**

$^1/_2$ **teaspoon onion powder**

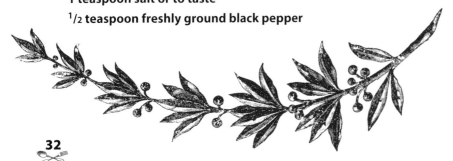

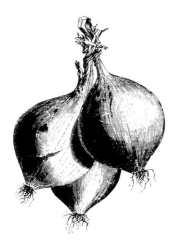

1. Combine the oil and vinegar, salt and pepper in a jar. Shake well until emulsified. The liquid should look slightly opaque, with the vinegar completely disbursed through the oil. If you are not using a jar to mix ingredients, put them in a bowl and beat with a fork or whisk to blend.
2. If you are adding other flavorings, toss them in the jar and shake again.

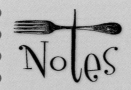

Notes

• If you are adding fresh herbs, you can combine them with the lettuce in the salad bowl or put them in the dressing before shaking. Most herbs blend beautifully together and you can use whatever you can get your hands on. Generally a combination of 2-3 herbs makes a nice mix (too many and you get a confusion of flavors). You can use a tablespoon of each for a large salad.

• A stick blender does a wonderful job of combining the dressing ingredients in a jar or tall-sided container.

• For a more pungent dressing, use only $^3/_4$ cup oil to the $^1/_4$ cup vinegar. If you are saving calories, you can add a little water to this mix, which will soften the vinegar flavor without adding more oil. Be sure to shake the mixture well before pouring since oil and water have a tendency to separate.

VERSATILE FRITTATAS

Frittata (frih-ta-ta) is a close cousin to the omelet, but it doesn't have that rarified air. Frittatas are simply scrambled eggs cooked with savory fillings. For an omelet, the filling is prepared separately from the eggs, then tucked into the pocket of cooked eggs flopped over on themselves. With the frittata, the filling is prepared in the pan and the eggs are poured over the filling. The two cook together, forming a homogenous whole. It can be slid from the pan and cut into slices like a pizza. The frittata bonus is lovely, crispy edges.

Frittatas aren't just for breakfast. Filled with meat, cheese and/or vegetables, frittatas make a wonderful light supper was well as a nourishing breakfast. Inexpensive and easy to prepare in a thousand variations, they make a great dish to serve to a crowd. They taste just as delicious at room temperature as they do hot.

I have seen a lot of recipes bandy the frittata name about, even when the dish is completely cooked in the oven. Cooked this way, the mixture puffs and becomes soufflé-like. An all-oven cooked frittata lacks the tasty crispy thinness that characterizes the best frittatas started on top of the stove.

The trick to cooking frittatas is to cook both sides without flipping the egg mixture. To do this, you first cook the eggs on top of the stove, heating from the bottom up. Next you move the eggs to the broiler, where they are cooked from the top down. Finishing under the broiler causes the eggs to puff just a little and turn golden, and preserves that crispy character around the edges. The eggs continue to cook as they sit on a cooling rack, so they should be slightly underdone when removed from the oven.

Some people prefer to cook a frittata completely on the stove top, which involves the much-dreaded flipping. To do this, you need a plate. When the bottom of the frittata sets up, slide it out of the pan and onto to the plate. Invert the mixture when sliding it back into the pan and finish cooking. This method scares me a little – too many ways to damage the lovely wholeness of the dish – which is why I prefer the oven finishing method. Frittatas cooked without the stint in the oven remain very thin, a characteristic some prefer.

My mom grew up eating frittatas; it is still one of her favorite dishes, especially when prepared with eggplant. Her recipe uses gently cooked onions and potatoes, flavored with a little olive oil and pepper. It is a vegetarian masterpiece, with familiar, homey flavors. But frittatas can be uptown too, with goat cheese, dill and smoked salmon, or roasted peppers, onions and Parmesan cheese. You can dress it up any way you want; the eggs will hold it all together and add the perfect complimentary flavor.

Frittatas can be made with whole eggs, or with one whole egg and egg whites. You could use an egg substitute if you are hell-bent on health, but I prefer the flavor of a real egg blended with whites. You can also add a splash of cream (or half-and-half) for richer texture and flavor. Otherwise, a little drizzle of water beaten into the eggs helps them froth up and lightens the dish. I like to figure on two eggs per serving, plus one for the pan. If going with egg whites, use one whole egg (the pan's, of course!) and then two egg whites per serving.

The great thing about frittatas is that the quantities are, if not irrelevant, then at least not an exact science. If you have an extra egg, throw it in. At the end of the cream carton? Toss it all in, too. If you want to use that leftover vegetable casserole, heat it up in the pan and throw in the eggs. If you have more filling than eggs, no worries; as long as you have enough liquid egg mixture to cover the surface of the filling, it will hold together. Or you can add a little extra cream to extend the eggs. Conversely, if you only have a little of a favorite ingredient, the frittata is a delicious way to make it go further; that last bit of gorgonzola cheese and smidge of pancetta, barely enough for one, expands to feed two (or more if you add a few other things like spinach, roasted peppers, maybe olives?) when encased in a frittata. No two frittatas are exactly alike, and that is a wonderful thing.

The filling for a frittata is a canvas for your creativity. Like pizza toppings, the fillings can go anywhere you want to take them. Only veggies? Veggies and cheese? Meat only? Meat and cheese? Meat, cheese and veggies? There are no rules, only Pepto-Bismol.

Some favorite combinations include mushrooms, onions and a white cheese like Monterey Jack, gouda, Swiss, provolone or mozzarella. Breakfast meats like sausage, ham or bacon can be paired with almost any cheese. Add a smidge of hash browns to the skillet and you have a complete meal in the pan. Roasted veggies (eggplant, onions, mushrooms, peppers, zucchini, asparagus, leeks) can be incorporated with a hearty sprinkle of cheese (try crumbled goat cheese). Diced salami or pepperoni and cheese can be paired, and then finished with a smear of olive tapenade on top of each slice.

BASIC FRITTATA

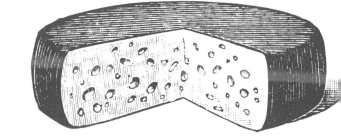

5 - 6 eggs

2 tablespoons cream or half-and-half

Salt and pepper to taste

1 cup of filling - a mix of meat, cheese, and/or vegetables

Olive oil and butter

1. Preheat the broiler.
2. Beat the eggs and cream, salt and pepper together and set aside.
3. Add a splash of olive oil and pat of butter to an oven-proof skillet. Heat on medium and add the filling ingredients except the cheese. Heat the ingredients thoroughly, stirring and spreading them evenly across the bottom of the skillet.
4. Pour the egg mixture over the filling, sprinkling with any cheese you are using.
5. Gently push the eggs towards the center of the skillet and let the liquid egg run out to the edges. Continue this moving until most of the eggs have formed curds but still are very wet, about 2 minutes. Continue cooking the eggs another 30 seconds without stirring.
6. Transfer the skillet to the broiler and heat until the top of the frittata puffs and turns golden, 3-4 minutes. Remove immediately and let sit for 1 or 2 minutes before slicing into wedges and serving. Garnish with a sprinkle of parsley or fresh herbs and a grind of pepper.

Serves 2

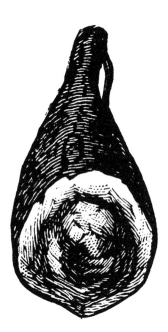

Filling suggestions – and the amounts are mere suggestions:
- **4 slices of bacon, $^1/_2$ cup of cheddar cheese**
- **$^1/_2$ cup roasted vegetable mix and $^1/_2$ cup Monterrey Jack cheese**
- **Small bunch of diced asparagus and $^1/_2$ cup Swiss cheese**
- **1-2 ounces goat cheese, fresh dill and slivers of smoked salmon**
- **Fresh tomatoes diced and drained - $^1/_2$ cup, chopped fresh basil, $^1/_4$ cup Parmesan cheese**
- **Sautéed onion, a handful of fresh spinach, and 1-2 slices crumbled pancetta**

RECIPES

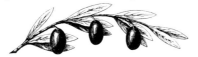

APPETIZERS

Dips and Spreads

Finger Food

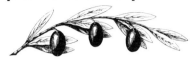
Layered Mexican Dip

So, this is one of those recipes that has been out there forever. Maybe longer. Yet, it continues to be one of the first empty dishes at a party or buffet. With layers of traditional Mexican flavors like seasoned meat, guacamole, tomatoes and cheese, each bite is a little different. It is always a huge hit with the teens, and is a terrific vegetarian option if you omit the ground beef. With its spectacular presentation, this baby will work at any tailgate.

1 pound ground beef

2 packages of taco seasoning

Optional: can of refried beans

8 ounces of sour cream

Guacamole

Salsa

Black olives

Chopped tomatoes

Green or red onions, chopped very fine

Fresh cilantro, loosely chopped (optional)

Sharp cheese grated, at least 2 cups, more to taste

Variety of corn chips

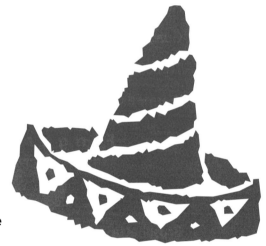

1. Brown the ground beef and season with one of the packets of taco seasoning. Add about half the package and taste. Add more if needed. Do not add the water as directed on the back of the package–you want the meat to be a bit dry.
2. Mix the other packet of taco seasoning with the sour cream.
3. On a large platter, spread first layer of beans and/or meat. This is your heaviest layer. You can combine the meat and beans in the skillet for a minute if you want, to really meld the two together, before spreading them on the platter.
4. Next add the seasoned sour cream layer. I always use this layer whether I have guacamole or not. Next add the guacamole.
5. Now start building layers of your choice: olives, tomatoes, onions, salsa.
6. End with cheese layer or make a pretty presentation by creating a design with colored ingredients: chopped green onions or olives in the middles, surrounded by tomatoes, surrounded by cheese to the edges.
7. Serve with colored corn chips – red, blue, white

Notes

•*This can be heated or served room temp. Tasty either way. If you want it heated, warm the meat and beans in the microwave until hot, then add your fresh ingredients.*

•*The ground beef can be drained on a paper towel before adding the seasoning mix to lower the fat in the dish.*

•*You could also make individual servings on small paper plates – a sort of super-nacho approach. Layer the chips down first, and then start adding the beans, meat, sauce, and garnishes.*

•*I love cilantro and always include it in anything Mexican. It is pretty chopped fine and sprinkled on top. Or include some in the guacamole or sour cream. If you are serving this to grade-schoolers, skip the cilantro.*

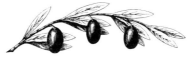

APPETIZERS

Dips and Spreads

• DIANE ROBBINS •

HOT CHEESE DIP

Diane is a wonderful cook who has an unerring instinct for crowd-pleasing recipes. This is one of her favorites. It makes a lot and keeps everyone happy when they visit her at the lake house. This is game-day fan food extraordinaire.

2 pounds Velveeta Cheese

1 8-ounce block cream cheese

1 pound mild sausage, crisply cooked, drained and crumbled

1 large jar (24 ounces) mild salsa (Pace Picante preferred)

1 can cream of mushroom soup

Corn chips

1. Mix together all ingredients except chips. Heat gently on the stove, or cook in the microwave in 1 minute intervals until all the ingredients are soft enough to combine.
2. Serve in a chafing dish or crock pot with chips.

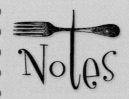

Notes

• *Velveeta gives the dip a smooth, homogenous texture. Its flavor is very mild. If you prefer a more robust cheese, use a sharp cheddar which you have shredded. You can even combine different cheeses, using half cheddar and half something else, like Monterey Jack, Pepper Jack, Havarti, Colby, or a white cheddar. Don't use a mild cheese like mozzarella or provolone; your dish will lack pizzazz.*

• *Diane uses Pace Picante salsa, but I enjoy trying different, exotic salsas of varying heat. Chipotles always figure in this somewhere at my house.*

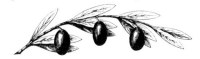

Dips and Spreads

Guacamole With Tomatillos

The addition of tomatillos to this recipe adds a refreshing, citrus-y lift to the flavor. It dilutes the richness of the avocado without compromising its distinctive flavor and feel. I also love the shortcut of adding salsa to get a quick hit of Mexican seasonings. The teenagers at my house adore this dish, and my son usually requests it when he comes home from college.

4-5 small to medium tomatillos

2 small avocados

2 green onions, white and pale green part of the stem, minced

$1/2$ cup sour cream

$1/4$ cup chipotle salsa, medium hot (or more, to taste)

2-3 tablespoons fresh cilantro, loosely chopped

Salt to taste

$1/2$ fresh lime

Chipotle chili powder (optional)

1. Remove the husks from the tomatillos. Bring a medium saucepan halfway filled with water to a boil. When the water reaches a rapid boil, drop the tomatillos in. Leave them for 1 minute, and then remove them to a bowl of ice water to stop their cooking.
2. Remove the core at the top with a paring knife, cutting away as little of the flesh as possible. Cut into quarters and place in the bowl of a food processor. Pulse a few times until the tomatillos are in very small chunks. Do not puree.
3. Pour the chopped tomatillos into a strainer set over the sink or a bowl and let the excess liquid drain off. If you skip this step, you will have very watery guacamole.
4. While the tomatillos are draining, slice the avocados in half; remove the pit and peel.
5. In a large, flat dish or shallow bowl, mash the avocado with a fork or pestle. Leave some small chunks. Sprinkle liberally with salt.
6. Add the tomatillos and onions to the avocado and blend. Fold in the sour cream and salsa next, then add the cilantro. Mix gently and taste for seasoning. Squeeze the lime over the mixture and blend.
7. If more heat is desired, sprinkle on some chipotle chili powder or add more salsa. Let the mixture sit a few minutes before serving to give the flavors a chance to marry. Serve as a dip with corn chips or as a relish/garnish to Mexican entrees.

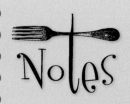

Notes

• *Tomatillos look like a small green tomato and usually are displayed near the tomatoes or with exotic ingredients like fresh ginger, fresh peppers, etc. in the grocery store. They have a husk whose freshness and greenness is a quality indicator. The husk must be removed. You should not substitute green tomatoes for the tomatillos in this dish. They are very different.*

• *A hand-held potato masher makes quick work of mashing the avocados.*

• *Yogurt can be substituted for the sour cream for a healthier version. Try using the wonderfully thick Greek yogurt if you can find it. It has superb tang and texture, very similar to sour cream without the guilt.*

• *If you want more heat without the smoky flavor, add a dash of cayenne pepper instead of the chipotle chili powder.*

• *Feel free to modify quantities of each ingredient. If you want to make the dish go further, add a little more sour cream and salsa. Beef up the number of tomatillos you use. Just be sure to taste for salt and lime juice after everything else has been added. You may want to add a little more cilantro, too. Play with it – no amount is hard and fast – all the flavors work well together in almost any proportion.*

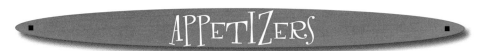
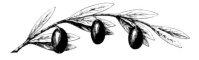

• **DIANE ROBBINS** •

Three Cheese Spread

Diane keeps this dip on hand in the summer to keep both the grandkids and adults happy. It is first cousin to pimento cheese.

8 ounces sour cream

2 cups (1 pint) Hellmann's mayonnaise

$^1/_2$ cup onion, minced

Sprinkle of garlic powder

Freshly ground black pepper

2 cups grated mozzarella cheese

2 cups grated cheddar cheese (mild or sharp)

6 tablespoons shredded Parmesan cheese

Assorted crackers

1. In a large bowl, blend the sour cream, mayonnaise, onion, garlic powder and pepper (to taste.)
2. Add the cheeses and blend well.
3. Serve with an assortment of crackers

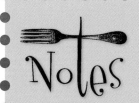

Notes

• *This will keep several weeks in the refrigerator.*
• *Be fearless with additions: jalapenos, Chipotle chili powder (about a teaspoon to begin with, more to taste) toasted nuts, a little chopped fresh rosemary*

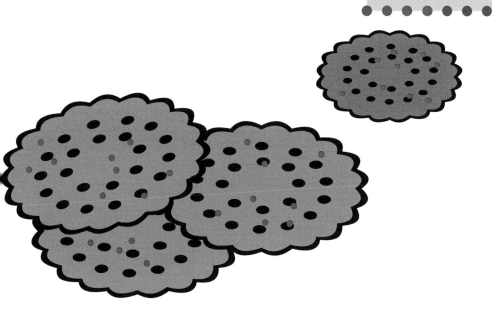

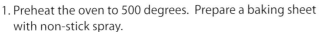

• KATHY HALL •

Warmed Cranberry Brie

OK, I know there are very few children in this world that will approach a runny Brie without saying "Ewww!" But the adults - ah, now that is a different story. They will crowd around this assertive cheese, warmed and dressed with cranberries and spice, sugar and rum. This fabulous appetizer would be great for a day of watching the sport of your choice on TV with a crowd. Or how about serving it at a Christmas party, surrounded with lots of green parsley as a garnish? Or maybe just fix it for yourself for dinner one night with a glass of wine. Who needs salad? Or guests?

1 16-ounce round brie

1 16-ounce can whole cranberry sauce

$^1/_4$ cup brown sugar, firmly packed

2 tablespoons spiced rum (or orange juice)

$^1/_2$ teaspoon ground nutmeg

$^1/_4$ cup chopped pecans, toasted

Toasted wheat crackers and apple slices

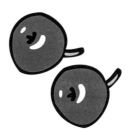

1. Preheat the oven to 500 degrees. Prepare a baking sheet with non-stick spray.
2. Carefully remove the top off the brie with a very sharp knife, leaving the rind around the sides as a border. Place the brie on the baking sheet.
3. Stir together the cranberries, sugar, rum or juice and nutmeg. Spread over the top of the brie.
4. Sprinkle with pecans and bake for 5 minutes or until softened and beginning to approach runny.
5. Serve with crackers and fruit.

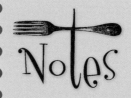

Notes

• *Pecans that have been toasted have a much richer flavor than untoasted pecans. It doesn't take long and is worth the effort. Since these pecans will be toasted a little in the oven while baking the dessert, they can be lightly toasted beforehand. To toast: put pecans in a heavy skillet over medium high heat. Watch carefully, and toss constantly as they begin to brown. Do not walk away from these while they are cooking or they will burn! Their high fat content helps them to brown very quickly.*

• *For a little kick, try adding a pinch (just a pinch!) of chipotle powder or cayenne pepper to the cranberry sauce mixture. The hit of heat activates another tasting spot on the tongue, and creates another layer of flavor. The contrast of the heat also enhances the sweetness and tartness of the mixture. Just a little dab will do ya!*

• *Pear slices are a lovely combination with brie and blend well with the cranberries.*

• *If you have an attractive serving utensil that can withstand the oven's high heat, use it. Life will be much simpler if you don't have to transfer the hot cheese from a baking sheet to a serving dish.*

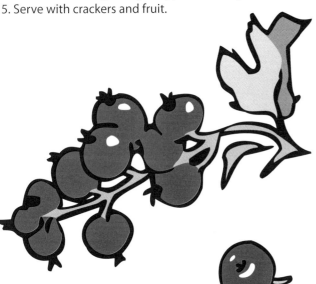

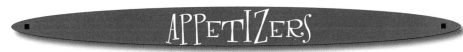

Finger Food

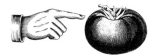

Bruschetta
(brew-sket-ta)

Authentic bruschetta is quite simple: thick slices of bread that have been toasted, brushed with a little high quality olive oil and rubbed with a clove of garlic. That's it; no cheese, no toppings. This recipe, although it is called bruschetta, is a distant cousin to what you would find in Italy. But it does have lots of Italian ingredients like olives, fresh tomatoes, basil and thick, crusty bread. It has a number of steps, each of which is easy. The toasts and toppings can be made the day before and assembled right before serving. Worth the effort! This crunchy, savory appetizer is a hit at every party it attends. It definitely is an adult pleaser.

Olive paste

    1 cup pitted ripe olives (Kalamatas are ideal)

    2 teaspoons balsamic vinegar

    1 teaspoon capers (try to find the dry ones preserved in salt rather than liquid)

    1 teaspoon high quality olive oil

    2 cloves garlic, minced

    1 8-ounce loaf crusty French bread (baguette)

    Olive oil

    $^1/_2$ cup freshly grated Parmesan cheese

Tomato Topper

    2 medium red and/or yellow tomatoes (1 cup), chopped

    $^1/_3$ cup thinly sliced green onion

    1 tablespoon olive oil

    1 tablespoon fresh snipped basil or oregano or 1 teaspoon dried basil or oregano leaves

    $^1/_4$ teaspoon fresh cracked pepper

    Salt to taste

1. For olive paste: process the olives, vinegar, capers, 1 teaspoon olive oil and garlic in a food processor until a nearly smooth paste forms. Cover and chill mixture for up to 2 days.

2. For the tomato topper: drain the chopped tomatoes before adding the other ingredients, otherwise the mixture will be too runny. Stir together the chopped tomatoes, green onion, 1 tablespoon olive oil, basil or oregano, salt and pepper. Cover and chill for up to 2 days.

3. For the toasts: Preheat the oven to 425 degrees. Slice bread on the diagonal into $^1/_2$-inch pieces. Brush both sides of each slice with olive oil and place on an ungreased baking sheet. Bake the toasts for 5 minutes until crisp and light brown. Cool and store in an airtight container for up to 24 hours.

4. To assemble: spread each toast with a thin layer of olive paste. Top with 2 tablespoons of tomato topper; sprinkle with Parmesan cheese. Bake at 425 degrees for 2-3 minutes until cheese starts to melt and the topping is heated through.

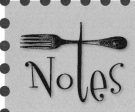

Notes

• *Use a good quality olive oil for this recipe – its flavor will shine through.*

• *Don't go near the Parmesan cheese in a can. Look in the deli department for freshly grated cheese, or buy a hunk and grate it yourself.*

• *This recipe doubles beautifully. And you probably can stretch your toppings to cover more than 24 rounds.*

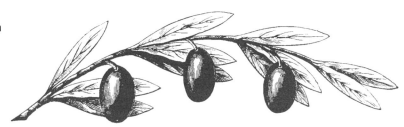

Makes about 2 dozen

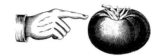

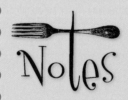

Cheddar Rosemary Dates

A friend who used to cater our office parties at the newspaper gave me this recipe years ago. It won't have the kids flocking to the table – but the adults and teenagers are a different story. No one is quite sure what it is before they bite into one of these, and they are even less sure after that first bite – but they love it. It is a fabulous mix of tastes: the sweetness of the date and the savory cheese flavor enlivened with fresh rosemary. The pecan is just icing on the cake. This is one of my most requested recipes.

1$^1/_2$ cups (6 ounces) shredded sharp Cheddar cheese

1 cup all-purpose flour

1 teaspoon salt

2 teaspoons chopped fresh rosemary

$^1/_3$ cup unsalted butter (6 tablespoons), melted

24 pitted dates (at least - see notes)

24 toasted pecan halves (at least – see notes)

1 egg white

Sugar

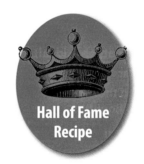

Hall of Fame Recipe

1. Preheat the oven to 350 degrees. Grease a baking sheet, or coat with non-stick spray.
2. Combine the cheese, flour, salt and rosemary, stirring well to mix. Add the butter and mix with a fork carefully, just until the dry ingredients are moistened. The dough will be quite crumbly, but it will hold together when pressed.
3. Make a lengthwise slit in each date and stuff with a pecan half.
4. Holding about 1 tablespoon of dough in your cupped hand, press the stuffed date into the center of it and work the dough around to completely cover the date. They should look like little cheese missiles. Cover and chill 1 hour. The dates can be frozen at this point, if desired. They will keep one month.
5. Place the dates on the baking sheet and brush with the egg white, which has been lightly beaten. Sprinkle with sugar.
6. Bake for 25 minutes. Remove to a rack to cool. These can be served warm or at room temperature.

Makes at least 24 – but can make quite a few more, depending on how thick the cheese dough is layered around the date.

Notes

• *Handle the dough gently so you don't toughen it. It presses rather easily around the date in spite of being crumbly.*

• *These are sensational warm – the date is kind of gooey and the cheese dough is crunchy. But they are equally tasty after they have cooled off, and continue their cheesy, crunchy goodness the next day. Pop one in the microwave for about 10 seconds for an instant replay.*

• *I find the dough always covers at least 30 dates (and usually more). These take some effort to make, so I try and get as many from the recipe as possible. If you prefer a very thick cheese covering, figure you will get closer to the 24 count.*

• *I would not substitute low fat cheese or margarine for butter. It is better to have one simply divine bite than four so-so nibbles.*

Finger Food

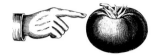

• CAROL POWELL •

Cheese Biscuits

My good friend, Carol, likes to give these biscuits as a Christmas gift to friends. She notes they contain all the elements needed for the perfect food: fat and crunch, nuts and cheese, sweet with a little zing of pepper. They make a lovely accompaniment to chicken salad, vegetable soup, or a platter of ham. Or fried chicken, or chili, or a hearty green salad. Or beside a crisp sausage patty and fried egg– well, you get the idea. . .

3 sticks of unsalted butter (1^1/2 cups), room temperature

1 pound of sharp cheddar cheese, grated

4 cups flour

1 teaspoon salt (optional, doesn't seem to need it)

Dash cayenne pepper (or use more if you like the zing!)

Pecan halves

Confectioner's sugar or large crystal brown sugar

1. Preheat the oven to 350 degrees. Line a cookie sheet with parchment paper or spray with non-stick spray.
2. Cream butter on medium speed of a mixer, beating until it lightens in color, about 4-5 minutes.
3. Add grated cheese, salt, cayenne pepper. Work the mixture until it is homogenized. Since you are not using any other liquid, you need to be sure your fat is evenly distributed. Use your hands for the most efficient blending. They will be getting messy when you add the flour anyway. You don't have to worry about toughness until you add the flour, so do a good job of blending at this point.
4. Work in the flour, starting with 2^1/2 cups. Work the dough as gently as possible to keep your biscuits tender. Add more flour gradually, but only enough to make a dough that holds together well and isn't too crumbly. You might not need the full 4 cups.
5. Roll dough to ^{1}/4 inch thickness and cut with a medium or small size cutter (see notes). Combine and re-roll dough after each cutting until all the dough has been cut. Handle gently.
6. Press a pecan half on each biscuit. Bake for 15 to 20 minutes.
7. Sprinkle with confectioner's sugar or large-crystal brown sugar while warm.

2 – 2 ^{1}/2 dozen medium biscuits

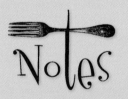

Notes

• *These tasty nuggets are best when cut into a smaller-than-standard size biscuit. They tend to be crumbly and fall apart when you bite them, so make them bite sized.*
• *The single pecan half looks lovely, but I like to use coarsely chopped pecans scattered on the top, too. It spreads out the toasty-nut flavor and is easier to bite than the whole piece.*
• *Be sure to use a nice, sharp cheese so the biscuits are not too bland.*
• *If you are going to use these as a savory accompaniment, eliminate the powdered sugar at the end.*

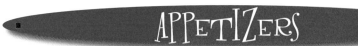
Finger Food

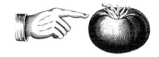

• MARY FAIRCLOTH AND JEANETTE REISENBURG •

CRISPY PARMESAN TOASTS

This is the simplest of recipes – and one of the best you'll ever eat. Crispy bread with a warm cheesy, herby spread is the perfect combination. Even my husband, who loathes mayonnaise, likes this. We had it for the first time while camping at Flat Creek Ranch in Jackson, Wyoming. Our host, Jeanette, fixed it in the cook's tent and we devoured it with great relish after a day of hiking. It is wonderful on a tapas menu, but it is great finger food, too, so it works well in a buffet, served at room temp – although warm is best. Older kids will love this one.

4 Pita rounds

1 cup Parmesan shredded cheese

$^1/_2$ cup mayonnaise

2 teaspoons Italian seasonings

1 teaspoon fresh lemon juice

Dash of cayenne (optional)

1. Preheat the oven to 375 degrees.
2. Combine the cheese, mayonnaise, Italian seasonings, lemon juice, and cayenne if using. Mix gently.
3. Spread $^1/_4$ of the mixture on each pita round.
4. Bake for 15 minutes until the cheese bubbles.
5. Cut into triangles and serve immediately.

Serves 4

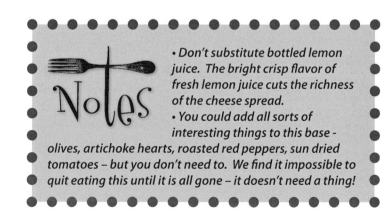

Notes

• *Don't substitute bottled lemon juice. The bright crisp flavor of fresh lemon juice cuts the richness of the cheese spread.*
• *You could add all sorts of interesting things to this base - olives, artichoke hearts, roasted red peppers, sun dried tomatoes – but you don't need to. We find it impossible to quit eating this until it is all gone – it doesn't need a thing!*

APPETIZERS

Finger Food

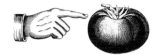

• RUBY HERRING •

FRIED BREAD

This is a beloved family recipe. My Louisiana grandmother would make a bagful for us to take in the car on our long ride home after a visit. She got up at dawn to fry it before we left. It smelled so good we would start eating it before we got down the driveway. Fried bread is a real crowd-pleaser. It is a simple recipe to make, but it takes a little time to fry the whole bag of bread dough. It incorporates all the important food groups: carbs, fats and sodium.

1 package frozen bread dough

4-6 cups olive oil (one large bottle or can)

Salt

1. Let the dough thaw and rise (*see Notes*). This will take several hours. When it has doubled in bulk, it is ready to fry.
2. Cut or tear the dough into bite-sized pieces. Shoot for an approximate size and shape of your pointer finger. Long and lean cooks faster than short and fat.
3. Pour all the olive oil into a heavy, deep skillet (a cast iron Dutch oven is perfect) that is at least 2 inches deep. Heat the oil over medium high heat until tiny bubbles form around the edge of the pan.
4. Drop a test piece of dough into the hot oil. If it rises immediately and is surrounded by bubbles, the oil is ready. If the dough sinks to the bottom of the pan and stays there, the oil is not hot enough. Wait another minute or two and test again.
5. Once the oil is hot enough, add dough pieces. They should have plenty of room to float around; don't crowd them. If you add too many at once, the oil will cool down and the dough will get soggy.
6. Cook until the dough on one side turns golden, about 3 minutes; flip and finish cooking until both sides are done. Monitor the oil temperature carefully. If the dough is browning too quickly, the inside will be raw while the outside is too dark.
7. Drain on a paper towel and sprinkle immediately with salt. Hold in a warming oven while the rest cook. Or put them on a platter and watch them disappear.

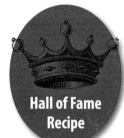

Hall of Fame Recipe

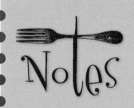

Notes

• *You can use frozen dough or make it from scratch. I have tried it both ways and can't tell a lick of difference between the two. My conclusion: it isn't worth the effort to make the dough from scratch.* Any brand of frozen dough works.

• *Don't waste your money on fine and fancy olive oils. Just use the large size from the grocery store.*

• *Thaw the bread overnight in the refrigerator if you plan ahead far enough. It will rise more than you thought possible. Make a slit or two in the bag to give the dough room to rise.*

• *If you like a lot of crust, tear the dough instead of cutting it. The irregular shapes will give you more surface area and result in a crispier, crustier piece.*

• *If you like your bread dough-y, make each piece nice and fat instead of long and lean.*

• *You could sprinkle the hot fried bread with sugar if you wanted a sweet treat, but nothing beats the salt!*

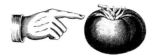

Finger Food

• **SHARON HERRING** •

SAVORY STUFFED MUSHROOMS

OK, so this is not one of those quick and easy, feeds-a-thousand-with-a-can-of-soup recipes. I have included it because it is just too darn good not too. My sister-in-law, Sharon, developed the recipe for these mushrooms in her California kitchen, and they are little bites of heaven. The mushroom makes the perfect envelope for a savory mixture of meat and a pesto-like paste full of herbs, cheese and nuts. A quick bake and you have a fabulous appetizer. This is definitely a grown-up flavor, great for a tailgate or buffet. If you stuffed large portabellas, a couple would make a lovely lunch-size serving. You could also make a vegetarian version without the meat.

8 large mushroom caps	one bunch basil
2 cloves garlic	2 tablespoons mint, chopped
one small onion	$^1/_4$ cup walnuts
$^1/_2$ red bell pepper	$^1/_4$ cup feta cheese
Olive oil	3 tablespoons freshly grated Parmesan cheese
$^1/_4$ pound ground turkey meat (or beef)	pinch of paprika (optional)
one bunch cilantro	salt and pepper to taste

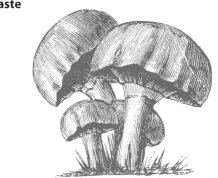

1. Preheat oven to 400 degrees.
2. Clean the mushroom caps with soft cloth. Snap off the stems and set them aside.
3. Finely chop onion, red bell pepper and garlic.
4. Add a dash of oil to a skillet or treat with non-stick spray. Heat until shimmering, then add the onions, pepper and garlic. After the vegetables cook down, about 3 minutes, add the ground meat. Cook until meat is browned. Salt lightly while it cooks. Be sure to crumble meat into small pieces while cooking. Remove mixture from the pan and drain on a paper towel.
6. Add the cilantro, basil, mint, walnuts, Feta cheese, Parmesan cheese and reserved mushroom stems into a food processor and pulse until mixed into a paste.
7. Combine the meat mixture with paste, stir well.
8. Stuff each mushroom cap with mixture.
9. Place stuffed caps on a cookie sheet and cover loosely with aluminum foil. Cook covered for 17 minutes, uncover and cook until mushrooms are tender, approx. 5-8 minutes. Serve hot.

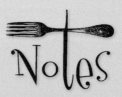

Notes

• *This recipe doubles easily – and in fact, eight measly mushrooms won't be enough when you and your guests get a taste. Just plan on doubling this.*

• *Use a nice, crumbly Feta that is packed in brine, and freshly grated Parmesan. Stay away from the green cans of cheese.*

• *Fresh herbs are critical to this dish – but you could fool around with them if you don't have the mint or basil. Try some fresh oregano, a snippet of chives, even a little rosemary if you have it.*

• *To keep the mushrooms from breaking when you stuff them, try microwaving them first. Spread them out on a plate and cook on High for 2 minutes, then turn them upside down on paper towels to drain them. Stuff as usual.*

RECIPES

BREAKFAST

Breakfast Dishes

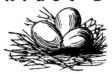

Breads

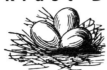

Breakfast Dishes

• PATTI PEARSON •

Baked fruit

This is a great side dish for a brunch, but kids go for it anytime. They love the spicy warm fruit topped with the crunchy oat topping. Try it as a dessert with a dollop of vanilla ice cream, whipped cream, or frozen yogurt.

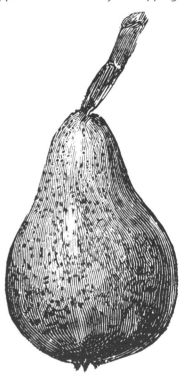

1 can (29-ounce) pear halves

1 can (29-ounce) peach halves

1 can (20-ounce) pineapple slices plus extra small can pineapple chunks

1 jar (10-ounce) maraschino cherries (optional)

1 cup sugar

2 tablespoons flour

$^1/_2$ teaspoon nutmeg

$^1/_2$ teaspoon cinnamon

$^1/_2$ cup rolled oats

$^1/_2$ cup flour

Dash salt

$^1/_2$ cup (1 stick) unsalted butter

$^1/_2$ cup orange juice

1. Preheat the oven to 350 degrees and butter a 9x13-inch dish.
2. Drain the pears, peaches, pineapples and cherries if using, and cut larger pieces in half.
3. Mix the fruit together and add the sugar, 2 tablespoons flour and spices.
4. Pour into the buttered dish.
5. Combine the oats and $^1/_2$ cup flour with a dash of salt and sprinkle over the fruit.
6. Melt the butter. Combine the orange juice and butter and pour the mixture over the fruit. Bake uncovered for 1 hour.

Serves 8

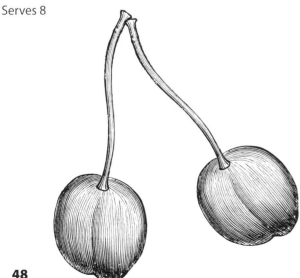

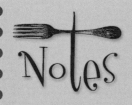

Notes

• *Coarsely chopped pecans or almonds could be added to the topping.*
• *This battle plan could work for any canned fruit – how about sour cherries and pineapple, and leave out the maraschino cherries? Or maybe a berry mix of canned blueberries, blackberries and cherries? Lots of options. Just combine your fruit of choice with flour, sugar and spices, add the topping and pour on the butter and juice.*

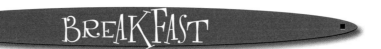
Breakfast Dishes

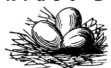

• MISSY HUTTON •

Spicy Breakfast Apples

These are delicious served with a sausage casserole or a grits casserole. Kids like apples, especially when they are sweeter than nature intended, like these. Try a splash of rich cream on top if you are serving them separately in a bowl. A good buffet dish.

$^1/_2$ **stick of butter (4 tablespoons)**

5 large apples, peeled, cored and sliced

1 cup brown sugar

1$^1/_2$ teaspoon cinnamon

$^1/_4$ **teaspoon nutmeg**

1. Melt butter in a large skillet over medium high heat. Add the apples and stir until well-coated with butter.
2. Add the sugar and spices and sauté until the apples are tender, about 15 minutes. If the mixture is too wet, continue cooking over low heat until the moisture evaporates. Serve warm.

Serves 4-6

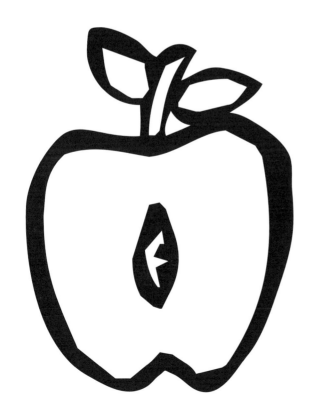

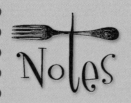

Notes

• *Granny Smith apples are perfect for this dish – they are not too sweet and are firm-textured. You could use other varieties like Gala, Fuji, or Pink Lady. I would avoid the red or golden Delicious varieties because they become mushy when cooked.*

• *Check for sweetness before serving – some apple varieties might need a little less or a little more sugar.*

• *Try adding $^1/_2$ cup raisins with the apples.*

• *You could substitute pears in this recipe for a delicious change.*

Breakfast Dishes

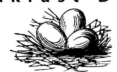

Blueberry French Toast

This is an incredibly rich treat, full of cream cheese and egg custard. The blueberries provide the perfect fruity counterpoint. Kids love it because syrup is involved. It makes a great buffet dish because it cooks up in large pans, can be made ahead, and tastes swell at room temperature. I first had it at a bed and breakfast outside of Asheville many years ago, and it has been my go-to recipe for overnight guests ever since.

1 loaf white bread (day old)

2 8-ounce loaves of cream cheese

1 cup blueberries (fresh or frozen)

12 eggs

2 cups milk

1/3 cup maple syrup or honey

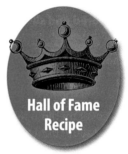

Hall of Fame Recipe

1. Lightly grease a 13x9x2-inch pan. Preheat the oven to 350 degrees.
2. Remove crusts from bread and tear or cut bread into 1-inch pieces. Place half the bread in the bottom of the pan.
3. Cut the cream cheese into 1-inch cubes and scatter half over the torn bread.
4. Sprinkle half the blueberries over the cream cheese.
5. Repeat layering the bread, cheese and berries.
6. Beat the eggs then add the milk and syrup, mixing well. Pour the egg mixture over the bread layers.
7. Cover and chill for 8 hours or overnight.
8. Remove the pan from the refrigerator 30 minutes before baking. Bake, covered, for 30 minutes at 350 degrees. Uncover and bake another 25-30 minutes or until the center is set and golden brown. Serve with Blueberry topping.

Serves 8 easily

Blueberry Topping

1 cup sugar

2 tablespoons cornstarch

1 cup water

1 cup blueberries (fresh or frozen)

1 tablespoon butter

1. Mix sugar and cornstarch together in a small pan. Add water. Bring to boil and boil for 3 minutes, stirring constantly.
2. Add the fruit, reduce heat and simmer 8-10 minutes or until the berries burst open. Stir in the butter. Serve warm over French Toast.

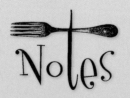

Notes

• *It is important the bread be really stale. Slice it and set it out in the air the night before to dry it out. It will now soak up the liquid without getting mushy.*
• *Any berry would work in this recipe: blueberry, strawberry, raspberry, boysenberry – let your pocketbook be your guide.*
• *Mrs.. Butterworth's Country Recipe syrup is good because it has vanilla and cinnamon in it for added flavor.*
• *For a healthier version, use low fat cream cheese and 2% milk.*
• *If using frozen berries in the syrup, you will need to cook it longer before the berries burst.*

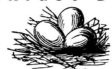

Breakfast Dishes

Oatmeal Casserole

This dish is perfect for a breakfast buffet. It feeds a bunch and is easy to make. It looks and sounds good for you – and it is! – but when you taste a spoonful you don't think about anything but how delicious it is. Blueberries spike the flavor of rich, creamy oatmeal baked in a casserole. Try serving it hot with a splash of cream or milk on top, just like you would a bowl of the best oatmeal you will ever eat.

2 cups frozen blueberries
2 tablespoons fresh lemon juice, divided
18 ounces (one container) regular oats
3 large eggs, beaten
1 cup brown sugar, packed firmly
1 cup unsweetened applesauce
1$^1/_2$ tablespoons ground cinnamon
$^1/_4$ teaspoon nutmeg
4 teaspoons baking powder
1 teaspoon salt
1$^1/_4$ cups water
1 cup milk
$^1/_4$ cup ($^1/_2$ stick) melted butter

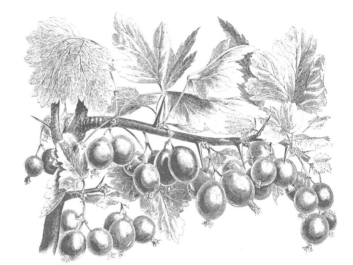

1. Preheat the oven to 350 degrees. Prepare a 9x13-inch pan with non-stick spray.
2. Toss the blueberries with 1 tablespoon of the lemon juice. Spread evenly on the bottom of the pan.
3. Combine the oats with the remaining ingredients and one tablespoon lemon juice. Spread evenly over the blueberries.
4. Bake, covered for 30 minutes. Uncover and continue baking for another 20 minutes, until the casserole turns golden brown and sets up.
5. Serve hot with cold milk or cream for pouring.

10-12 servings

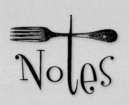

Notes
• Fresh blueberries work as well as frozen.
• Try using different firm fruits: apples, peaches, cherries, pears.
• Nuts are a great addition. Spread $^1/_2$ - 1 cup of chopped nuts over the fruit before adding the oatmeal. Pecans, almonds, or cashews would work beautifully. Try toasting them for 5 minutes in a skillet before baking. The toasting really brings out the nutty flavor.

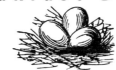

BREAKFAST

Breakfast Dishes

• KATHY HALL •

Overnight Breakfast Casserole

This recipe is an old standard that never gets old. It requires an overnight sit for the bread to soak up the egg mixture. It puffs up as it bakes, so you have a savory filling of cheese and sausage surrounded by a fluffy, egg custard. Only really young kids might be timid about eating this, but once they taste the cheese and sausage, they relax. Tell 'em it tastes like a Sausage McMuffin (only better!) This holds well at room temperature, making it a winner for the buffet table. Leave out the sausage and you have a vegetarian dish.

1 pound ground pork sausage

10 white sandwich bread slices, cubed (6 cups)

8 ounces (2 cups) shredded sharp cheddar cheese

6 large eggs

2 cups milk

1 teaspoon salt

1 teaspoon dry mustard

$^1/_4$ teaspoon Worcestershire sauce

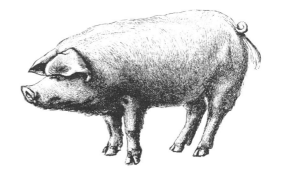

1. Brown sausage over medium heat, breaking it up as it cooks. Drain on a paper towel.
2. Treat a 13x9-inch baking dish with grease or non-stick spray. Arrange bread cubes in a layer on the bottom of the dish. Sprinkle with cheese; top with sausage.
3. Whisk together eggs, milk, salt, mustard and Worcestershire sauce; pour evenly over the sausage-cheese mixture.
4. Cover and chill the casserole 8 hours or overnight.
5. The next day, preheat the oven to 350 degrees and bring the casserole out of refrigeration. Let it sit for 30 minutes to bring it up to room temperature.
6. Bake for 45 minutes, or until set.

Serves 8

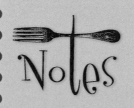

Notes

• *The original recipe calls for white bread. Spread your wings and try something with a little more body (but not too much!) Thinly sliced French or Italian bread works well. You could even use herbed bread, like rosemary focaccia, if you wanted to dress it up.*
• *The drier your bread, the better this recipe works. Consider leaving whatever bread you use sitting out overnight to dry out. It will soak up the egg mixture better without disintegrating.*
• *You could use different meats with this - bacon, ham, kielbasa, flavored chicken sausage – for an interesting variation.*

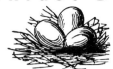

Potato and Egg Bake

This is a rich, one-dish casserole that has everything in one little pan: potatoes, cheese, ham and eggs. Oh – and a stick of butter! It is perfect for breakfast, but it could also be appear on the dinner table with fresh fruit and sourdough bread. Leave out the meat, and you have a great vegetarian entrée, or a delicious side dish. It can also be made the day before and reheated before serving. I might add that it is delicious right out of the fridge, unheated.

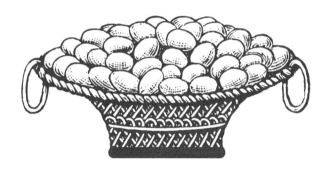

¹/₂ cup butter (1 stick)

1 16-ounce package frozen hash browns

1 cup cheddar cheese, shredded

2 cups Swiss cheese, shredded

2 cups diced ham or browned, crumbled sausage

5 eggs

1 cup milk

Chopped onions to taste (optional) about 1 cup

1. Preheat the oven to 450. Melt butter in a 9x13-inch pan.
2. Add hash browns to the pan and toss to coat with the butter. Bake at 425 degrees for 30 minutes. Remove from the oven and lower the temperature to 350.
3. While the potatoes are baking, beat together the eggs and milk and add the cheddar and Swiss cheeses, meat, and chopped onions. Pour the mixture over the browned potatoes.
4. Bake for 30 minutes. Let stand for 5 minutes before cutting.

Serves 6-8

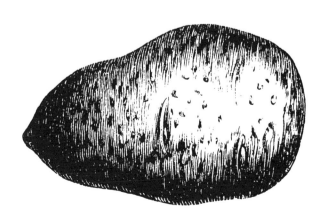

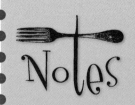

Notes

• *My family likes a little more sausage in this one than just the one pound. We also like the hot variety. You could use a variety of meats other than breakfast sausage, like Italian sausage, Kielbasa, or turkey sausage.*
• *Play with cheese combinations – or just a single cheese for all 3 cups.*
• *The onions lend a distinctive flavor. If you are serving this to younger kids, leave them out.*
• *For a robust variation, throw in some chopped jalapenos and a teaspoon of chipotle chili powder (mix with the eggs and milk.) Ole!*

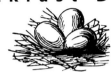
Roasted Chile and Egg Bake

This is a spectacular breakfast/brunch option. Creamy with four different cheeses, spiced with mild chile peppers, it has a wonderful custard texture that is soothing for the first meal of the day. The first time I had it at a bed and breakfast in the Napa Valley, it was served with link sausage, sourdough bread and homemade preserves. This feeds a crowd easily. It is not spicy – just flavorful.

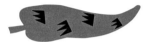

For 4 -6 servings

    5 eggs

    $^3/_4$ cups ricotta cheese

    $^1/_4$ cup small curd cottage cheese

    $^1/_4$ pound (4 ounces) grated Sonoma Jack cheese

    $^1/_4$ pound (4 ounces) grated sharp cheddar cheese

    1 7-ounce can fire-roasted chiles

    2 tablespoons diced jalapeno peppers

    $^1/_2$ teaspoon baking powder

    $^1/_4$ cup flour

    $^1/_4$ teaspoon salt

    $^1/_4$ cup ($^1/_2$ stick) unsalted butter, melted

    Grated Parmesan cheese

1. Preheat the oven to 350 degrees. Grease a 9x13-inch pan.
2. Beat eggs until light and lemon colored. Add cheeses and diced peppers.
3. Sift together dry ingredients and add very slowly. Stir in the melted butter.
4. Pour into the well-greased pan. Sprinkle with Parmesan cheese.
5. Bake 45 - 60 minutes until top is lightly browned.

Recipe for 20:

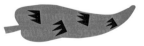

    20 eggs

    3 cups Ricotta

    1 cup small curd cottage cheese

    1 pound (16 ounces) grated Sonoma Jack cheese

    1 pound (16 ounces) grated sharp cheddar

    3 7-ounce cans fire-roasted diced chiles

    4-ounce can diced jalapeno peppers

    2 teaspoons baking powder

    1 cup flour

    $^1/_4$ teaspoon salt

    1 cup (2 sticks) unsalted butter, melted

    Grated Reggiano Parmesan cheese

1. Follow directions at left, preparing two pans. If you want the dish to be creamier, use a pan or casserole smaller and deeper than 9 x13.

Notes

• *Fire-roasted chiles can be tricky to find. Check the olive/relish section of the supermarket, and look for them in a glass jar. Also check the gourmet section. The roasted flavor adds so much to the final product; it is worth seeking out the chiles. If all else fails, substitute regular diced green chiles. Melissas.com carries its own brand of fire roasted chiles you can order online.*

• *You can roast your own chiles if you want. Use 2-3 mild fresh chiles like Anaheim and broil them close to the element, turning occasionally until all sides have turned black. Wrap the hot chiles in a paper towel or tuck into a zip-top bag. Let them sit for about ten minutes and then peel; the skin will come off easily. Remove the stem and seeds, chop and add to the recipe. For the smaller quantity, start with one chile, adding more as taste dictates. Be sure to keep your hands away from your eyes while you are handling the chiles.*

• *Sure, you can make this lower fat with reduced fat cottage and ricotta cheeses, and reduced fat cheddar. I would avoid the non-fat variety, though. The flavor and texture will change too much. You can cut back on the amount of butter, but don't eliminate it.*

• *Use the finest Parmesan on top you can, since it provides a sharp contrast to the creamy concoction below. Steer clear of anything that comes in a can. Check the deli department for pre-shredded or grated, high quality cheese.*

• *A tip for eggs: Crack them on a flat surface rather than a counter edge or bowl rim. The sharp edges drive the shell up into the egg.*

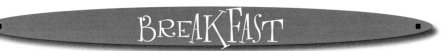

Breakfast Dishes

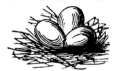

Sweet and Hot Bacon

This is an easy, delicious way to prepare a lot of bacon for a crowd. The salty, sweet and hot combination of flavors will get you going in the morning. Pair it with a mild, creamy breakfast casserole, like the chile bake, and fluffy hot biscuits with homemade jam.

Bacon

Chipotle chili powder

Dark brown sugar

1. Pre-heat oven to broil. Stretch bacon out in a single layer in a broiler pan.
2. Sprinkle the chili powder like you were salting the bacon for a nice, medium hot effect. Add more to taste. Sprinkle the brown sugar liberally on each slice.
3. Set the oven rack on the second rung from the top so the pan does not get too close to the element. Broil until crispy, turning once and adding more spice and sugar on the flip side if desired.

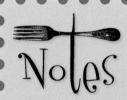

Notes

- *If you are using the same pan for several batches of bacon, be sure to drain the grease that accumulates between batches or you will have a mess and the smoke alarm will go off. Don't ask how I know.*
- *If you want to avoid the whole broiler situation, fry the bacon in a skillet but remove it before it becomes really crisp. It can start to brown, but it should still be fairly limp. The goal is to get most of the fat rendered. Spread the partially cooked bacon on a shallow baking sheet and sprinkle with sugar and chile. Bake in a 300 degree oven until crisp. Start checking after about 10 minutes. The baking enables the seasonings to sit on the bacon and soak in rather than leech away during the frying process.*

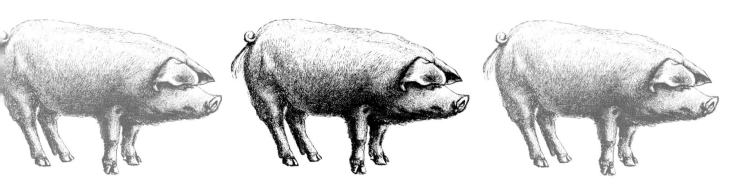

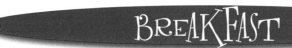

BreakFast

B r e a d s

• JACKIE JARVIS JONES •

Caramel Coffee Cake (sticky buns)

This is a great recipe for brunch. Sweet and gooey, with the crunch of pecans, it uses the convenience of frozen yeast rolls. Prepared the night before, the rolls will rise and be ready to go first thing in the morning. Pair with ham or bacon and a fresh fruit medley topped with minted yogurt, and you have a memorable meal.

1 bag frozen Parker House-style rolls

1 box butterscotch pudding mix (NOT instant)

1 cup pecans, chopped fine

$^3/_4$ cup brown sugar

$^3/_4$ cup butter (1$^1/_2$ sticks)

1. Spray a tube pan with non-stick spray. Place the FROZEN rolls in the pan. Sprinkle with the dry pudding mix and pecans.
2. Combine the brown sugar and butter in a small saucepan and bring to a boil over medium heat. Pour the mixture over the rolls and cover loosely with foil.
3. Leave the pan out on a counter overnight. In the morning, preheat the oven to 350 and bake the rolls for 30 minutes, uncovered.
4. Place the foil underneath the pan to catch any spills.

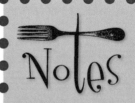

Notes

• *Be sure you get the right frozen bread – you want the rolls and not buns or other varieties. You will end up with a dry product if you grab the wrong thing from the freezer case. Been there, done that.*

• *This would be good using frozen biscuits, too. You will skip the overnight step and just pour on the flavored ingredients just before popping them in the oven. Just don't cook them too long. Check the package instructions for the appropriate baking time for the frozen biscuits.*

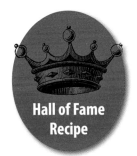

Hall of Fame Recipe

Cream Cheese Braids

I have made these as gifts for neighbors and office buddies for years. They are now an expected ritual at my house each Christmas. I usually make more than one batch – they are an impressive gift for someone for whom you just don't know what to buy – hairdresser, teacher, secretary. They are a gift of love for those you cherish. They are beyond fabulous. A sweet yeast dough encases a warm, runny cream cheese filling. The egg in the bread seems to make the braids lose their freshness quickly - but they never last long enough to get stale. The dough must rise overnight, and it must rise again the next morning, so plan ahead.

1 cup sour cream

$^1/_2$ cup sugar

1 teaspoon salt

$^1/_2$ cup (1 stick) melted butter

2 packages dry yeast

$^1/_2$ cup warm water

2 eggs, room temperature, beaten

4 cups all-purpose flour

Cream cheese filling

Glaze

Cream Cheese Filling

2 8-ounce packages cream cheese, softened

$^3/_4$ cup sugar

1 egg, beaten

$^1/_8$ teaspoon salt

2 teaspoons vanilla extract

1. Combine sugar and cheese in a small bowl.
2. Add egg, salt, and vanilla, mix well.

Yield: about 2 cups

Glaze

2 cups powdered sugar, sifted

4 tablespoons milk

2 teaspoons vanilla extract

1. Combine all ingredients and mix well. Thin with more milk if too thick. It should pour fairly easily. It will thin out from the heat when it is poured on the warm loaves.

Yield: about 1 cup

---

1. Heat sour cream over low heat; stir in sugar, salt and butter; cool to lukewarm.
2. Sprinkle yeast over warm water in a large bowl, stirring until yeast dissolves. (Note: I add a little sugar to the water to proof the yeast and make sure it is active – the mixture should foam up within a minute.)
3. Add cooled sour cream mixture and eggs to the yeast. Begin adding the flour in one cup increments, mixing well after each addition. The dough will be very sticky, even after all the flour has been added. Cover tightly; refrigerate overnight. Make sure the bowl you use is large enough to accommodate the rising of the bread.
4. The next day, punch the dough down and divide the dough into 4 equal parts. Roll out one part on a well-floured board into a 12 x 8-inch rectangle. Add a little flour if you need to keep the dough from sticking.
5. Spread $^1/_4$ of Cream Cheese Filling (about $^1/_2$ cup) on the dough rectangle, spreading the mixture almost to the edge; leave about $^1/_4$-inch border. Roll up jelly roll fashion, starting from a long side. Pinch edges together at the end and cut off excess if there is a lot. Fold under the ends; place, seam-side down, on a greased cookie sheet. Repeat with remaining dough and filling.
6. Slit each roll at 2-inch intervals in alternating angles about $^2/_3$ way through dough to resemble a braid. Be careful not to cut through too deeply.
7. Cover and let the loaves rise in a warm, draft-free place until doubled in bulk – about an hour.
8. Bake at 375 for 12-15 minutes (watch closely!).
9. Spread with Glaze while still warm.

Makes 4 loaves with very short shelf life

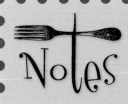

Notes

• *You can fit 2 loaves per cookie sheet if you don't mind the sides touching after they rise.*
It takes about 3 hours on the second day to make the bread; gift while still warm.
• *Use a really large bowl for dough to rise in - it gets huge.*
• *Use real vanilla extract, not imitation.*
• *If you have a non-stick pastry mat, use it for rolling out this sticky dough.*

Breads

• LEAH MOIR •

Healthy Bran Muffins

These big 'ol muffins are portable, healthy and tasty. They are the perfect "trunk food," as one friend says. She always kept a load of snacks in the trunk for her kids to eat en route from school to a practice or game. Chock full of fruit and nuts, sweetened with Splenda and applesauce, and enhanced with bran cereal, they take care of business before a game or early morning event – although with all that bran, I sure wouldn't serve them the day before a big event! These also make a great after-school snack, or between-game snack. Try them sitting out for overnight guests or on a breakfast buffet.

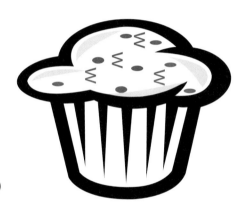

4 eggs

³/₄ cup Splenda or other sugar substitute

¹/₂ cup vegetable oil

1 cup buttermilk

1 16-ounce jar unsweetened applesauce

3 cups Kellogg's bran buds

1 cup raisins

1 cup finely chopped nuts

1 cup finely chopped cooking apples – about 1 large (skin on is fine)

1 cup whole wheat flour

1 cup whole bran flour

5 teaspoons baking powder

1 teaspoon salt

1. Preheat the oven to 350. Spray muffin tin with non-stick spray.
2. In a large bowl, combine the eggs, Splenda, oil, buttermilk, applesauce, bran buds, raisins, nuts and apples. Mix thoroughly and let stand for about 30 minutes.
3. Sift together the flours, baking powder and salt. Add the dry ingredients to the wet mixture and blend thoroughly, making sure to leave no pockets of unincorporated flour.
4. Spoon into the prepared muffin tin and bake for 25 minutes or until a toothpick comes out cleanly.

Yield: 24 large muffins

Notes

• *Toast the nuts before adding them to the recipe. Put them in a heavy skillet over medium high heat and cook for about five minutes, watching carefully so they don't burn. They will have a much deeper flavor in the muffins.*
• *I use unbleached flour for both the bran and wheat flours if that is all I have on hand. It makes a lighter, less dense muffin, equally delicious, less cleansing.*
• *Try mixing up the dried fruit a bit. One of my favorite substitutes is cranraisins. You could use dried blueberries, dried cranberries, dried cherries, dates, or prunes.*
• *The apples and applesauce are very important – no substitutes for the best results. The applesauce adds moisture and sweetness so you don't need as much oil and sugar. The chopped apple adds texture and moisture. I like to leave the skin on the apple for its nutrition and fiber – but with all that bran, if you prefer your apples peeled, you don't need to worry!*
• *One teaspoon of salt doesn't seem like much for this large a batch, but the cereal has sodium in it, so the amount is fine.*

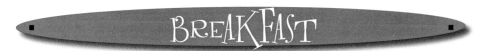

• MARY CONSTANTINE •

Pecan Biscuit Ring

This recipe was contributed by our local newspaper's food writer, Mary Constantine. Mary has a knack for putting together flavorful recipes that don't require a cooking school degree. This one is a great candidate for holiday morning breakfasts. Sugar, butter, biscuits – it won't just be kids who swoon over this one.

1 stick butter

1 cup chopped pecans

1 cup brown sugar

$^1/_4$ cup maple flavored syrup

2 cans extra-large size refrigerated biscuits

1. Preheat oven to 350 degrees. Coat a 12-cup fluted tube pan with cooking spray.
2. In a small saucepan over medium heat, melt the butter and stir in nuts, brown sugar and syrup. Mix well.
3. Pour $^1/_4$ cup syrup mixture evenly around the bottom of the pan. Add the biscuits, standing them on edge evenly around the pan.
4. Pour the remaining syrup mixture over the biscuits.
5. Place the pan on a baking sheet to catch any overflow and bake for 40 minutes.
6. Cool the bread for 3 minutes, then invert onto a serving platter. Serve warm or at room temperature.

Serves 6-8

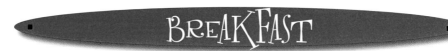

• KATHY HALL •

Sausage Cheese Muffins

A family favorite at Kathy's house, these make a delicious quick breakfast. Good travel food, they can also be thrown in a backpack. They are equally welcome at a buffet. These are a little rich for a pre-game meal, unless you have a few hours before the game. They couldn't be easier!

3 cups baking mix (for example, Bisquick)
1 pound sausage, cooked and crumbled
1^1/$_2$ cups shredded cheese
1 can cheddar cheese soup
^{3}/$_4$ cup water

1. Preheat oven to 375 degrees. Prepare muffin cups with non-stick spray.
2. Mix all ingredients and spoon into muffin cups.
3. Bake 25 minutes.

Makes 15 muffins

RECIPES

ENTRÉES

BEEF

CHICKEN

SEAFOOD

BEEF

• LEAH MOIR •

BASIC BEEF NOODLE CASSEROLE

Kid friendly, mom friendly, wallet friendly! Variation friendly, too! This is a simple dish with simple flavors: noodles, ground beef, tomatoes, and a mild cream sauce. It is a simple sort of beef stroganoff. Kids really go for it. Good for all ages and perfect for the buffet table when you have a crowd to feed.

1 pound ground round

1 8-ounce container of sour cream

1 can cream of mushroom soup

1 small jar of mushrooms

1 14-ounce can of diced tomatoes

1 package of egg noodles

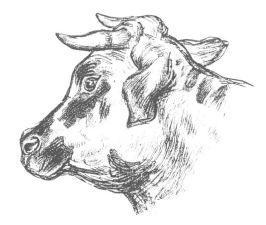

1. Preheat oven to 350 degrees. Prepare a large casserole with non-stick spray.
2. Start heating a large pot of salted water for cooking the noodles, using amounts on the back of the package of noodles.
3. Cook ground beef in a large skillet until browned, breaking it up into smaller pieces. Remove to a paper towel and blot thoroughly.
4. Combine sour cream, cream of mushroom soup, mushrooms and diced tomatoes in a large bowl.
5. Add the drained ground beef.
6. Cook noodles as directed on the package. Drain. Add the noodles to the ground beef mixture and pour into a casserole dish.
7. Cook uncovered until bubbly, about 30 minutes.

Serves 6-8

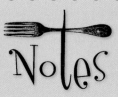

Notes

• *This is a good starting point for many variations. You could substitute stew beef for the ground meat. Or how about some chicken sausage in one of the myriad flavors offered? Or kielbasa sausage. You get the idea! The sauce components are neutral enough to work with almost any meat.*
• *To up the adult quotient, use fresh portabella mushrooms sautéed in butter instead of the jarred mushrooms. Slice 8 ounces of mushrooms and sauté in 2 tablespoons of butter.*
• *To give it an Italian vibe, use ground meat and/or Italian sausage and add some dried Italian seasonings to the sauce – about 1 teaspoon. You could also sauté some onions and garlic (1 onion, 2 garlic cloves) with the fresh mushrooms in some olive oil. Finish with a sprinkle of freshly grated Parmesan cheese.*
• *I like to use Rotel tomatoes instead of plain tomatoes for the heat and flavor.*
• *This dish could easily be topped with cheddar cheese or Parmesan cheese. Or both! Shred enough to cover the surface of the casserole, at least one cup or more, depending on the shape of your dish.*
• *More veggies? Throw in some peas, peas 'n carrots, broccoli, roasted peppers - most any veggie would work.*

B E E F

• **MISSY HUTTON** •

CASSEROLE Spaghetti

Boys love this casserole. It is a neater version of spaghetti, embellished with cheese and olives. Missy fixed it for her son's basketball team, and one of the boys said he wished there was a perfume that smelled like this. As a cook, it just doesn't get any better than that! Serve this with a crisp salad, some hot garlic rolls and a big, gooey brownie.

1¹/₂ pounds ground chuck

1 green bell pepper, chopped

1 large onion, chopped

¹/₂ cup celery, chopped

2 cloves of garlic, crushed

1 can cream of mushroom soup

³/₄ cup water or broth

1 16-ounce can of tomatoes, undrained and chopped

2 tablespoons chili powder

1 teaspoon Italian seasoning

¹/₂ teaspoon salt

¹/₄ teaspoon pepper

1 8-ounce package spaghetti, uncooked

2 ounces sharp cheddar cheese, cut into small cubes

1 5-ounce jar pimiento-stuffed olives, drained

³/₄ cup (3 ounces) shredded sharp cheddar cheese

1. Brown the chuck in a large skillet, stirring until the meat crumbles. As the fat renders, add the pepper, onion, celery and garlic. Cook until the vegetables are soft, around five minutes. Drain the mixture and return to skillet.
2. Stir in soup, water, tomatoes, chili powder, Italian seasoning, salt and pepper and bring to a boil. Cover, reduce heat and simmer for 1 hour.
3. Preheat the oven to 325 degrees. Lightly grease an 11x7-inch baking dish.
4. Cook spaghetti (see Perfect Pasta for tips on cooking noodles). Drain.
5. In a very large bowl, combine the cooked spaghetti, cubed cheese and olives, and meat sauce. Spoon into the prepared baking dish.
6. Cover and bake for 20 minutes, or until thoroughly heated. Remove from oven, cover with shredded cheese and cook uncovered an additional 10 minutes, until cheese is melted.

6-8 servings

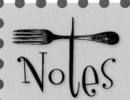

Notes

• *If fixing this for young kids, eliminate the olives*
• *If fixing for adults, try different olives, like a spicy black Greek olive. And add some sautéed mushrooms for even more flavor. Portabella would be wonderful. Sauté 8 ounces of sliced mushrooms in 2 tablespoons of butter.*
• *Try a different cheese for the topping, like a nice, gooey mozzarella or provolone mixed with the cheddar. And Parmesan is always good.*

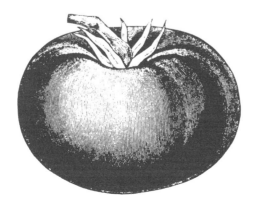

ENTRÉES

B E E F

• JOHN MULLANEY •

Comfort Lasagna

The first bite of this lasagna elicits a moment of reverent silence. It has been described as "slap yo mama" good. It may be the pesto-like cream sauce that dresses up each serving. Or the four cheeses. Or the Portobello mushrooms. One taste and you won't care; you'll just want more. This recipe comes from John Mullaney, associate pastor at Vestavia Hills UMC in Birmingham, Alabama. It is his much-anticipated signature dish he prepares for parishioners recovering from surgery or some other hardship. I don't doubt people step off curbs just to get a pan of this lasagna while they nurse their injuries.

1 red bell pepper, chopped

1 green bell pepper, chopped

1 onion, chopped

5 cloves of garlic, peeled and minced

Olive oil

1 8-ounce package sliced baby Portobello mushrooms

1 16-ounce package hot Italian turkey sausage with casings removed

1 medium can tomato sauce

1 small can tomato paste

1 cup red wine (the rest is for you)

2 cups water or broth

2 teaspoons garlic salt

2 teaspoons cayenne pepper

2 teaspoons black pepper

2 teaspoons chili powder

3 tablespoons (or more) fresh basil, chopped fine, divided

3 tablespoons (or more) fresh oregano, chopped fine, divided

1 container cottage cheese (full fat variety)

1 egg, beaten

1 package of no boil lasagna noodles

8 ounces mozzarella cheese, shredded

8 ounces fontina cheese, shredded

8 ounces sharp provolone cheese, shredded

1 cup Parmesan cheese, shredded

Basil Cream Sauce (recipe right)

1. Cover the bottom of a very large skillet with a thin layer of olive oil. When it is hot, add the bell peppers and onion. Cook 4-5 minutes, until the vegetables soften and turn golden.
2. Add the sausage and cook until browned, crumbling with a spoon. Drain off the fat if desired. (John leaves it in "for added awesomeness.")
3. Add the sliced mushrooms and cook 2-3 minutes until they begin to release moisture. Add the garlic and cook another minute or so.
4. Add the tomato sauce, tomato paste, wine, and 2 cups water or broth. Season with garlic salt, pepper, cayenne, and chili powder. Throw in the fresh basil and oregano to taste and stir to combine.
5. Let the sauce cook down for about 30 minutes (or until the bottle of wine is gone). Add more water as needed, or cook longer to thicken the sauce to desired consistency.
6. Preheat the oven to 350 degrees. Treat a deep 9x13-inch baking dish with non-stick spray.
7. Combine the four shredded cheeses and set aside.
8. In a bowl, mix the cottage cheese with the beaten egg. Add some fresh basil and oregano to taste.
9. Begin the layering process. In the bottom of the baking dish, start with:
   A layer of meat sauce
   Then a layer of noodles
   Then a layer of cottage cheese
   Then a layer of mixed cheese
10. Repeat the layers until the dish is full, ending with a cheese layer. Remember, THIN LAYERS WORK BEST.
11. Cover the dish with tin foil and bake for 30 minutes. Remove the foil and bake for 30 more minutes until the cheese is golden and bubbly.
12. Let the lasagna sit for 10 minutes to rest before serving. Drizzle each serving with Basil Cream Sauce and garnish with a sprig of fresh herbs.

Serves 10-12

64

continued on page 65

continued from page 64

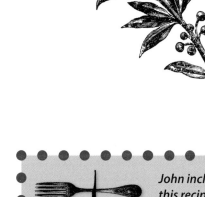

Basil Cream Sauce

> **Large bunch fresh basil (2-3 cups)**
>
> **Large bunch fresh oregano (2-3 cups)**
>
> **3-4 cloves garlic, minced**
>
> **$^1/_2$ cup Parmesan cheese, shredded**
>
> **Salt and pepper to taste**
>
> **1 tablespoon olive oil**
>
> **3-5 tablespoons of half and half**
>
> **Water (to right consistency)**

1. Combine the herbs, garlic, cheese, salt and pepper in a food processor. Pulse until completely mixed.
2. Add the olive oil and half and half and pulse a few times. Gradually add water to create a thin-ish sauce. Go carefully. If the sauce gets too thin, add some Parmesan to thicken it up. Or throw in a little butter.

Notes

John includes his own notes with this recipe. I pass them along.
- Don't get caught up in the measurements. Add what you like, in the amounts you like.
- Giving this lasagna heat is what makes it great, so hot sausage is a must.
- Give the sauce's ingredients time to mingle and get to know one another. That's what the rest of the bottle of wine is for.
- Don't underestimate the power of the Basil Cream Sauce.

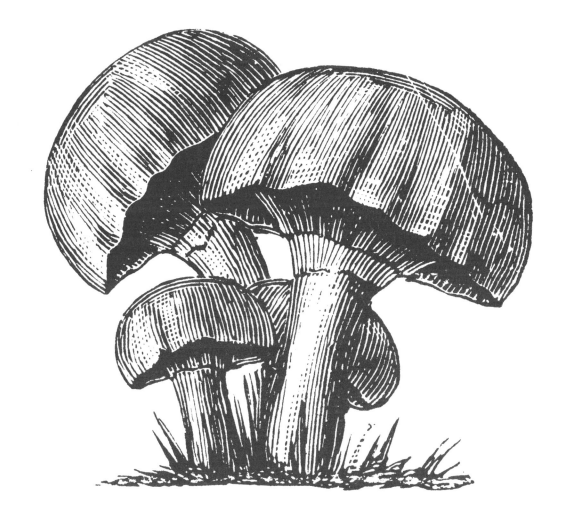

• LEAH MOIR •

Layered Hamburger Casserole

OK, this is one of those easy ones that kids love. Nothing exotic here, just favorite familiar flavors like tomatoes, noodles and cheese, layered like a lasagna. Pick fun shaped pasta – wagon wheels or bow-ties - the kids will love it, and it will be easier to eat than long, sauce-flinging noodles.

2 tablespoons butter or olive oil

1^1/$_2$ pound ground beef – a mix of ground chuck and sirloin

4 cloves garlic, minced

1 teaspoon salt

^{1}/$_2$ teaspoon pepper

2 (8-ounce) cans tomato sauce

1 (8-ounce) package flat noodles

1 (3-ounce) package cream cheese

1 (8-ounce) carton sour cream

^{1}/$_2$ cup grated cheddar cheese

1. Preheat oven to 350 degrees. Grease a casserole dish lightly with butter or treat with non-stick spray.
2. Melt butter. Toss in meat and cook until brown.
3. Add garlic to the meat, along with salt, pepper and tomato sauce. Cook 15 to 20 minutes.
4. While the meat sauce is simmering, cook noodles (see Perfect Pasta for tips on cooking pasta). Drain.
5. Mix softened cream cheese and sour cream.
6. Put a layer of noodles in the bottom of the greased casserole. Spread about ^{1}/$_3$ cheese and cream mixture, then ^{1}/$_3$ meat mixture. Repeat layers of noodles, cream mixture and meat mixture until casserole is filled. Sprinkle cheddar cheese over top.
7. Bake 15 to 25 minutes or until quite bubbly.

Serves 6

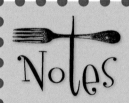

Notes

• *Ground chuck has more fat and flavor than ground sirloin, so I like to use a mix of both. Try a pound of sirloin and a half pound chuck for a lean version.*
• *Sure, substitute ground turkey and lower fat sour cream and cream cheese.*
• *Leave out the meat for a vegetarian tomato-ey mac 'n cheese.*
• *Add stuff for the adults: chopped onions, peppers, mushrooms. Cook in the meat drippings and combine with the meat when layering.*
• *How about a little Italian seasoning mix? 1-2 teaspoons should do it.*
• *A little Parmesan on top with the cheddar?*

• MISSY HUTTON •

Sausage Mac & Cheese Casserole

Even though this has breakfast sausage in it, this makes a great dinner. It is one recipe that has been around for a long time. It's like mac and cheese with sausage. An easy dinner, it works well in the buffet line. Perfect for a team meal. And yes, kids will eat it.

1 pound of mild breakfast sausage (Wampler brand recommended)

1 7-ounce box macaroni

1 can cream of celery soup

1 can cheddar cheese soup

1 large can Carnation evaporated milk

8 ounces mild cheddar cheese, shredded

Salt and pepper to taste

1. Preheat the oven to 325 degrees. Treat a large casserole dish with non-stick spray.
2. Brown the sausage in a heavy skillet. Break it up into small pieces while it is cooking. Drain on a paper towel.
3. Bring a large pot of salted water to a boil. Add macaroni and cook until al dente. Check the back of the macaroni package for recommended cooking time and subtract 2 minutes. The macaroni will get a second cooking in the oven, so it should not be overcooked at this point. Drain into a colander.
4. In a large bowl, combine the browned sausage, cooked pasta, cheddar and celery soups, and the evaporated milk. Taste for seasoning (you shouldn't need to add much salt since the soups contain salt already). Pour into the prepared casserole dish.
5. Sprinkle the mixture with the shredded cheese and bake uncovered for 30 minutes.

Serves 6-8

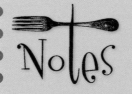

Notes

• *This dish starts out pretty safe with the seasonings, but it would be easy to kick it up. Use hot sausage and $1/2$ teaspoon chipotle chili powder (or more to taste.) You can also add about $1/3$ cup smoky salsa for an "Ole!" effect.*

• *A can of Rotel tomatoes adds another heated variation. Tomatoes significantly change this dish's personality – delicious but not as much of a mac 'n cheese vibe. Drain the tomatoes before adding them to the mixture so things don't get too wet.*

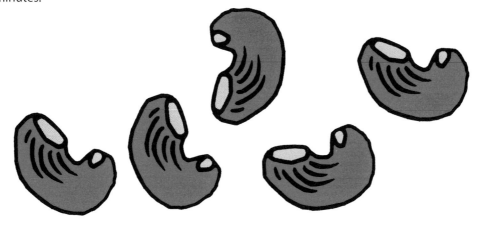

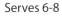

BEEF

• JOAN JORDAN •

Tagliarini

This is a delicious complete meal in a pan. Easier than lasagna, it has a similar sensibility with the addition of corn and olives. If you are serving kids, make sure the mushrooms are finely chopped, and consider eliminating the olives if the kids are really young.

1 pound ground beef

¹/₂ pound pork sausage

1 green pepper, chopped

1 onion, chopped

1 teaspoon garlic powder

1 can cream style corn

1 small can tomato paste

1 tablespoon Worcestershire sauce

1 tablespoon salt

1 teaspoon pepper

1 teaspoon hot sauce

1 tablespoon sugar

¹/₂ to 1 cup black olives, chopped

1 jar sliced mushrooms

1 package medium egg noodles, cooked and drained

Shredded cheddar cheese (4 ounces or more to taste)

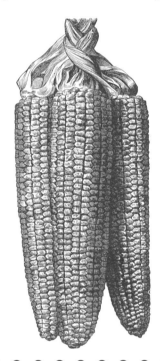

1. Preheat the oven to 375 degrees. Prepare a large casserole with non-stick spray.
2. Brown the meat and drain on a paper towel.
3. Cook the pepper, onion and garlic powder in the residue left from browning the meat until soft, about 5 minutes.
4. In a large bowl, combine the meat and the vegetable mixture. In another bowl, combine the corn, tomato paste, Worcestershire sauce, salt, pepper, hot sauce, sugar, olives and mushrooms. Mix well.
5. Pour the seasoning mixture over the meat and add with the noodles. Spoon into the prepared casserole dish. Bake uncovered for 35 minutes.
6. Top with cheese and run under the broiler until the cheese melts, about 5 minutes – but watch closely.

Serves 6-8

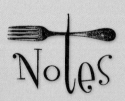

Notes

• *Sugar? It balances the acid in the tomatoes. You don't have to use it, but it rounds out the flavor.*
• *Try fresh mushrooms (I always go for the Portobellas because of their big flavor) sauteed in a little butter or added to the peppers and onions cooked in the pan juices.*
• *You could use mozzarella cheese instead of cheddar. If you do, try adding about ¹/₃ cup Parmesan cheese blended with the mozzarella. It adds a wonderful sharp accent.*

BEEF

•LEAH MOIR•

Cowpuncher Beef and Rice

This recipe doubles easily and is a cinch to make. It freezes well, too. Make several and have them in the freezer for a quick fix during the weeknight. Or be ready for that phone call for a covered dish at school or church. This recipe can be safe, with limited seasoning, or wild with more chili powder and peppers. Either way, the combination of rice, beef and tomatoes topped with cheese is a real crowd pleaser. This is a good one for the kids.

1 pound lean ground beef (or a mix of chuck and lean)

1 teaspoon jalapeno pepper sauce

1 small green pepper, chopped

1 small onion, chopped

1 large clove garlic, minced

$^1/_2$ teaspoon chili powder, plain or chipotle

$^1/_2$ teaspoon dry mustard

$^1/_2$ teaspoon dried whole oregano

1 teaspoon salt

1 15-ounce can stewed tomatoes

2 cups cooked regular rice

$^1/_2$ cup shredded cheddar cheese

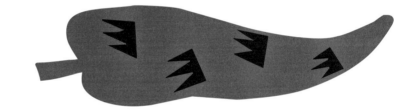

1. Preheat the oven to 350 degrees. Grease a $1^1/_2$ quart casserole.
2. Brown the ground beef with some salt and the pepper sauce. Remove and drain on a paper towel. Sauté the garlic, green pepper, and onion in the beef drippings until soft, about 5 minutes. Drain on a paper towel.
3. Combine the tomatoes, chili powder, dry mustard, and oregano in a large bowl. Add the rice and meat mixture. Stir gently until uniformly mixed. Check seasoning. Turn into the prepared casserole.
4. Cover and bake for 30 minutes; add the shredded cheese and bake, uncovered, an additional 10 minutes or until the cheese is nice and bubbly but not browned.

Serves 6

Notes

• *Use whole canned tomatoes and chop them yourself with an immersion blender or a quick spin in the food processor. Or simply squeeze them with your hands to break them up as you add them to the pot. Whole tomatoes have a better flavor and fewer additives than the diced variety. I prefer Muir Organic. Fire-roasted is especially good.*
• *Ready for some heat? Add some jalapenos, both in the body of the casserole and sprinkled on top with the cheese. Or use a mixture of cheddar and pepper jack cheese on top.*
• *Feeling crazy? Use a can of Rotel tomatoes instead of plain old tomatoes. And, you can always increase the amount of chili powder to up to one tablespoon. Taste as you go.*

BEEF

• LEAH MOIR •

Mini Empanadas

These are just too good not to make sometime. They are labor intensive, as is any food prepared in individual servings, but really pretty simple - and so delicious! Kids go nuts for them – cute little nuggets of meaty/cheesy goodness they can carry around and eat without a fork. They are good at room temperature, so they could be packed in a box dinner for after the game.

1 package refrigerated pie dough in large sheets

1 pound ground beef

1 cup thick and chunky salsa

1 can sliced ripe olives

1 cup shredded Mexican cheese blend

All-purpose flour for dusting

1. Preheat oven to 400 degrees.
2. Brown ground beef in a large skillet on medium high heat. Drain well, patting with paper towels to remove as much grease as possible. Return to the skillet and combine with salsa and olives. Bring the mixture to a boil, then reduce heat and simmer for 5 minutes. Check seasoning. Remove from heat and stir in cheese.
3. Roll dough out on a flour dusted surface. With a 3-inch round cutter, cut out 18 circles, re-rolling scraps as needed. Place about 1 tablespoon of the beef mixture in the center of each circle. Moisten edges with water. Fold circles in half and pinch to seal. Pierce tops with fork.
4. Place empanadas on baking sheet. Bake for 15 minutes or until golden. Serve hot.

Makes 1¹/₂ dozen

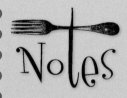

Notes

• *Canned olives are easy, but fresh deli olives add so much more flavor. Look for a pitted variety – ripe or green, both are good.*
• *I like to add the cheese separately from the meat filling – just a sprinkle on top of the filling before you close up the empanada.*
• *Naturally, you can experiment with fillings. Try chopped cooked chicken mixed with some cream cheese, green chiles and pepper jack cheese.*
• *Plain old breakfast sausage browned and combined with cheddar cheese would be a winner, too! I'm of the opinion that anything encased in pie dough is going to taste pretty darn good.*
• *Go Italian and use Italian sausage and mozzarella or provolone cheese. You could even put a scant teaspoon of prepared spaghetti sauce in each empanada before folding up and sealing. Maybe a sprinkle of Parmesan?*

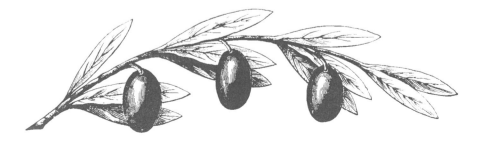

BEEF

• MISSY HUTTON •

Sloppy Joes

Kids love these. Sloppy Joes just taste like home. They are messy to eat, but you can bet they WILL be eaten. Try and use the freshest buns possible - it makes such a difference! Or serve the meat mixture over baked potatoes with a sprinkle of cheddar cheese.

1^1/$_2$ pounds ground beef

^{1}/$_2$ teaspoon garlic powder

^{1}/$_2$ teaspoon onion powder

1 14-ounce can pureed tomatoes

1 6-ounce can tomato sauce

Salt and pepper to taste

1 tablespoon Worcestershire sauce

1 teaspoon sugar

1 teaspoon vinegar

Chili powder to taste

Serves 6-8

1. Brown beef, season with salt, pepper, onion powder and garlic powder as it cooks. Drain the beef.
2. Combine cooked beef with remaining ingredients and simmer. Serve over the freshest hamburger buns.

Notes

- *If you like a stronger sweet/sour character, up the sugar and vinegar amounts to a tablespoon each.*
- *I usually use about a teaspoon of chili powder, but you may want to taste as you go and add the seasoning gradually.*

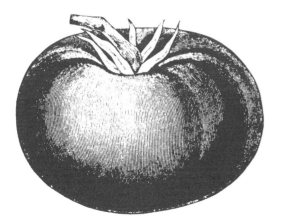

BEEF

•CINDY BAIRD•

Stromboli

Meat and cheese, rolled up in fresh dough and baked until it is hot and gooey - this is a favorite of all ages. Sublime served hot, Stromboli is also quite tasty at room temperature, which makes it a great choice for food on the bus after a game with chips, fruit and a cookie. Cindy says this recipe serves six to eight – or one boy!

1 loaf frozen white bread, thawed

Pepperoni slices

Salami slices

Ham slices or other luncheon meats

1 8-ounce package Mozzarella (pre-shredded is OK)

1 egg, beaten

1. Pre-heat the oven to 350 degrees.
2. Roll out bread dough in a rectangle as thin as possible. Cover the surface of the bread by placing the pepperoni, salami and ham in rows. Top with cheese.
3. Starting from the long side, roll like jelly roll and tuck under the sides.
4. Bake 20 minutes in 350 degree oven. Remove and coat with 1 beaten egg. Bake 5 to 10 minutes longer.
5. Slice and serve.

6-8 servings

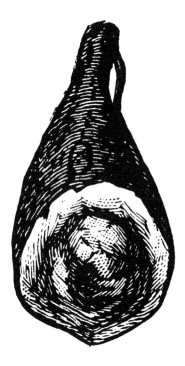

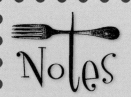

Notes

• *Try using turkey versions of the meats for a low-fat variation.*
• *Add some grated Parmesan cheese for extra kick.*
• *For a crispier Stromboli, slice it before baking. Eliminate the egg wash and watch for browning after 15 minutes.*
• *All sorts of additions are possible with this recipe: olive salad for a mufaletta variation, or pizza-type veggies like mushrooms, peppers, onions – sauté them lightly before adding to the Stromboli; don't forget the jalapenos!*
• *You could turn any of your favorite sandwich combinations into Stromboli. Just layer them in the dough, roll and bake. Try a Reuben version with corned beef, Swiss and kraut; a club with turkey and bacon; a vegetarian with spinach and herbed soft cheese, maybe some strips of red pepper or sun dried tomatoes; roast beef, provolone and sautéed onions and peppers; sliced steak and blue cheese; maybe some barbecued chicken and extra sauce. Anything baked inside the bread is going to be tasty!*

B E E F

• PAM MULLINS •

Tamale Pie

This dish appeared frequently on the family table when I was growing up. I can remember my mom stirring the big pot of meat and cornmeal while the wonderful smell filled the kitchen. This is a great party dish – inexpensive and filling. The flavors are classic: ground beef, chili, corn and cheese, baked in an easy-to-serve casserole. It can be as mild or spicy as you want. The amounts used below produce a medium/spicy dish that will scare away only the pathologically timid. This is a great make-ahead dish that freezes well. Serve with a crisp green salad dressed with a sharp vinaigrette, guacamole, and a chocolate dessert.

1 pound ground chuck or ground round

1 tablespoon olive or canola oil

1 onion, chopped

4 cloves of garlic

2 16-ounce cans tomato sauce

1 large can of whole kernel corn, drained

2 tablespoons chili powder (use more or less to taste)

1 teaspoon cumin

1 teaspoon chipotle chili powder (optional)

Salt and pepper to taste

1 cup milk

1 cup yellow cornmeal

1 – 1$\frac{1}{2}$ cups grated Parmesan cheese

Optional: 1 small can chopped black olives

1. Preheat the oven to 350 degrees. Prepare a large casserole dish with non-stick spray.
2. Brown beef in a large skillet with high sides until the meat is browned, crumbly and fairly dry. Season with salt and pepper while cooking. Remove meat to a paper towel and drain.
3. In the same skillet, add oil if not enough fat was rendered from the cooked meat, and sauté the garlic and onions until soft and fragrant, 6-8 minutes. Return the meat to the pan.
4. Add the tomato sauce, corn, chili powder, chipotle chili powder if using and cumin to the pan. Stir to blend evenly. Taste for saltiness.
5. Add the milk and cornmeal to the skillet and cook gently for 10 minutes, stirring constantly. This will make a thick, heavy mixture.
6. Put the mixture in the prepared casserole dish and spread Parmesan cheese $\frac{1}{4}$ inch thick on the top. Pat down firmly. Sprinkle with the chopped black olives.
7. Bake at 350 for 30 – 40 minutes until bubbly and cooked through.

8-10 servings

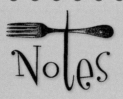

Notes

• Omit the olives if making this for kids – they will probably just pick them out. If you want a memorable dish, try using a strongly flavored olive, like a Kalamata olive. You could even use a mixture of green and black olives, although the pies of my youth were always prepared with mild canned black olives.

• Ground turkey can be used instead of beef. If using turkey, sprinkle with some of the chili powders and cumin, as well as salt and pepper, while browning. Also, since turkey is so lean, spray the pan with non-stick spray or add a little oil to the bottom of the skillet before browning.

• The Parmesan cheese adds a wonderful bite to the dish, but you could use other cheeses, too. A mild white queso would be delicious grated on top. Or an assertive Pepper Jack. Or a nice, sharp cheddar. Try a mixture of cheeses if you are feeling a little crazy! • Whichever cheese you choose, use enough to create a nice blanket completely covering the casserole below.

• Loosely chopped cilantro and a squeeze of fresh lime juice make lovely finishers.

BEEF

• LEAH MOIR •

Texas Shepherd's Pie

This is a great kid dish. Sneaky vegetable alert! Most kids won't notice the veggies in the sauce – they'll be too excited about the mashed potatoes. The potatoes are mashed with buttermilk, which gives them a tangy personality that holds up well to all the other flavors in the pie. The fennel seed gives it an intriguing but not too foreign flavor. This is an excellent buffet item – unusual and always popular.

1^1/$_2$ **pounds (2 medium) peeled baking potatoes - cut into ^{1}/$_4$-inch thick slices**

^{1}/$_3$ **cup low-fat buttermilk**

1 teaspoon salt - divided

^{1}/$_2$ **teaspoon white pepper - divided**

1 pound ground round

^{1}/$_2$ **cup chopped onion**

^{1}/$_3$ **cup chopped celery**

^{1}/$_4$ **cup shredded carrot**

^{1}/$_2$ **teaspoon fennel seeds - crushed**

1 teaspoon instant minced garlic (or fresh, if preferred)

1^1/$_2$ **cups salsa (1 16-ounce jar)**

Cooking spray

^{1}/$_2$ **cup (2 ounces) shredded regular or reduced-fat sharp cheddar cheese**

1. Preheat oven to 375 degrees. Treat an 8x8-inch baking pan with non-stick spray.
2. Place potato slices in a medium saucepan. Cover with water; bring to a boil. Reduce heat, and simmer, uncovered, 10 minutes or until tender; drain. Return potato slices to pan and cook over low heat until all the moisture has evaporated.
3. Add buttermilk, ^{1}/$_2$ teaspoon salt, and ^{1}/$_4$ teaspoon pepper; beat at medium speed of a mixer until smooth. Set aside.
4. Cook the meat in a large nonstick skillet over medium-high heat until browned, stirring to crumble; drain.
5. Return meat to pan. Add ^{1}/$_2$ teaspoon salt, ^{1}/$_4$ teaspoon pepper, onion, celery, carrot, fennel seeds, and garlic; cook over medium heat 5 minutes or until vegetables are crisp-tender, stirring frequently.
6. Add salsa; simmer over medium-low heat 10 minutes. Taste and correct seasoning.
7. Spoon into the baking dish; spread potato mixture over meat mixture. Sprinkle with cheese.
8. Bake, uncovered for 20 minutes or until thoroughly heated.

4-6 servings

Notes

- *Add more cheese to the topping if you want. Or try using a pre-shredded, three-cheese Mexican blend.*
- *If you use fresh garlic, mince it finely and cook with the beef as you brown it.*
- *My favorite salsa is Chipotle Salsa. It has a medium heat and a wonderful, smoky flavor. Vary the heat of the dish by the heat of the salsa you use. I like to use hot, because it gets pretty diluted with all the other ingredients, but for a younger crowd, I would definitely go mild.*

Cheesy Meatballs

These moist and meaty balls can be served in a crusty roll topped with pasta sauce and cheese, or over pasta with extra sauce. They are so flavorful, they can make even store-bought spaghetti sauce taste homemade. Adding the cheese to the meat mixture gives the meatballs a delicious richness.

1 pound ground beef

$^1/_2$ pound ground pork

1 egg, lightly beaten

3 cloves garlic, minced

1-2 tablespoons chopped Italian parsley

$^1/_2$ medium yellow onion, chopped extremely fine

2 teaspoons Italian seasoning (or more to taste)

$^1/_3$ cup freshly grated Parmesan cheese

Italian bread crumbs

Salt and pepper to taste

Pinch of cayenne

2 tablespoons olive oil

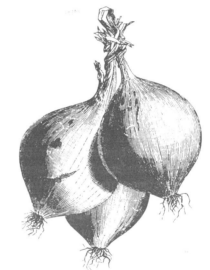

1. In a large bowl, gently blend the two meats with your hands.
2. Add the egg, garlic, parsley, chopped onion, Italian seasoning and Parmesan cheese, salt, and pepper; mix thoroughly but gently with your hands. Add enough bread crumbs (start with $^1/_4$ cup) to make a firm, but still moist, mixture. If you add too much, just throw in another egg to loosen it up.
3. Pinch off a little bit of the mixture and cook it quickly in a little oil heated in a heavy skillet. Taste and correct seasoning.
4. Shape the mixture into small balls – about the size of a giant olive – if using for sandwiches. The meatballs can be larger if they are going into a pasta sauce.
5. Roll the mixture firmly between your hands until it's no longer crumbly, but handle the meat gently.
6. Heat a little more olive oil in the skillet. When the oil is hot, add the meatballs, being careful not to crowd them. Brown on all sides. Remove and drain on paper towels. Add more oil as needed while browning the rest of the meatballs.
7. Serve with jarred or homemade marinara sauce, or nestle into rolls for meatball sandwiches.

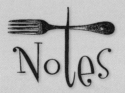

Notes

• *If you'd like, use Italian sausage instead of ground pork. Just remove it from the casing before mixing. Your finished product will be spicier (not hotter). You could also substitute breakfast sausage, hot or mild, for the ground pork.*

• *If you don't have any breadcrumbs on hand, pulverize some salad croutons in a processor. You'll get the body you are looking for plus a big flavor boost.*

6-8 servings

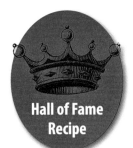

Hall of Fame Recipe

BEEF

• RUBY HERRING •

Nana's Garlic Brisket

This is THE number one crowd-pleasing recipe in my entire collection. Fall-apart tender and infused with garlic, it fills your house with the most inviting, incredible aroma. I have fixed it for groups countless times, and there never is any left. I have to make copies of this recipe every time I serve it. The baseball boys asked for it every year. It is good for tailgating, picnics, neighborhood dinners – it feeds a crowd without breaking the bank. It is easy to fix, but a bit messy to cut since you are working with such a large piece of meat. Worth every bit of trouble!

**1 large vacuum-sealed beef brisket
(8 pounds and up – do NOT use anything smaller)**

**1 package dried onion soup mix
(I like Knorr, less salty than Lipton)**

6-8 cloves of garlic (or more, to taste), peeled and slivered
Freshly ground black pepper
Dash of chipotle chili powder (optional)
1 -2 packages kielbasa or polish sausage

1. Trim the fat on the top of the brisket down to about $^1/_4$ inch. You need to leave some fat to keep the beef moist during the long, slow cooking. You can have the butcher trim the fat for you if you can't face all that fat, but in my experience they usually take off too much. You have better control if you just take a sharp knife at home and go at it.

2. Flip the brisket over to the non-fat side. Make deep slits all over with a small knife and stuff with slivers of garlic. The slits should be about 2 to 3 inches apart. Don't worry about too much garlic – can't happen! Push the garlic all the way in so it is deep inside the meat.

3. Flip the brisket over again, fat side up. Place in a large pan with deep sides since brisket will render a lot of juice.

4. Sprinkle the brisket with the dried onion soup mix, pressing mixture into the fat. Grind some black pepper on top. Lots of it. Sprinkle on the chipotle chili if using.

5. Cover the pan with tinfoil and place in a 275-degree oven. Forget the meat for about 5 hours. Remove the foil and begin basting the meat infrequently for the remaining cooking time. You may need to remove some of the accumulated liquid. Or, if you removed a little too much fat in step one, you may need to add a bit of water.

6. Place the polish sausage or kielbasa around the beef and continue cooking the brisket for at least another 3 hours, more is fine (I have cooked them for as long as 12 hours.)

7. Let the brisket cool about $^1/_2$ hour before slicing. Cut across the grain for the least amount of shredding (although the "shreds" make wonderful sandwiches.)

8. Strain the drippings, which will contain a lot of fat. Return the juices to a medium pan and heat.

9. Make a slurry of about 2 tablespoons of flour thinned with water. It should pour easily. Be sure to mash out any lumps in the flour with the back of a spoon before adding to the drippings.

10. Slowly add the slurry to the gently boiling juices, stirring constantly. Continue to stir and cook over medium heat until the gravy thickens nicely. Taste for seasoning. You probably won't need much salt since the soup mix is already salted.

11. Serve the brisket with gravy and horseradish sauce. Slice the sausage on the diagonal and serve alongside the brisket with spicy mustard.

Serves 8-10 easily

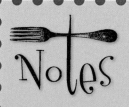

Notes

• *It is crucial to use a large brisket – do not use the tip that has been trimmed down to 3-4 pounds. It will dry out and be inedible. I usually use one in the 12-15 pound range. The bigger the better. You can freeze any leftovers.*

• *Brisket freezes beautifully, or it can be made 2-3 days ahead and kept in the fridge. If holding in fridge, simply slice cooled meat then arrange in your oven-proof dish. Drizzle liberally with gravy and press plastic wrap across the surface. Seal the dish with tinfoil and refrigerate. Reheat slowly the day you want to serve in a 275 oven for 2-3 hours. Be sure to remove the plastic wrap before reheating, but keep the dish covered with tin foil during reheating.*

Flank Steak Pinwheels

This is an easy way to make an inexpensive and healthy cut of meat as elegant as fine steak. Melting tender and full of flavor, these pinwheels are perfect for company. Serve with Crispy Parmesan Toasts and a fresh salad. Try them for your next grill-out – great for tailgating!

2 – 2¹/2 pounds flank steak
Bottled marinade
Toothpicks

1. Two to three hours before you are ready to grill, pull the flank steak from the refrigerator. Treat the meat with a meat tenderizer that pierces the meat to tenderize it. If you don't have one, use the tip of a sharp knife and pierce the meat every few inches, or stab with the tines of a fork.
2. Place the meat in a large zip top bag and pour in the marinade, using the amount recommended on the bottle. Zip up and refrigerate for 2-3 hours.
3. While the grill is warming up, pull the meat from the refrigerator and let most of the marinade drip off in the sink. Lay the meat on a clean, flat surface. Starting on the long side, roll up the meat, jelly-roll fashion.
4. With the seam side down so the roll doesn't open back out, slice off one-inch slices and secure with a toothpick.
5. Let the meat sit until it comes up to room temperature, about 20 minutes; don't put cold meat on the grill.
6. Grill pinwheels 6 minutes on each side for medium rare.
7. Let the meat sit for 5-10 minutes before serving to let the juices settle back into the meat from the surface.

Serves 6

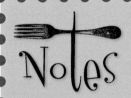

Notes

• My marinade of choice is Thomas Marinade, a blend of oil, vinegar, and soy sauce, with herbs and other flavorings. Annie's Naturals also has some wonderful marinades. Experiment with different styles - Japanese, South American – any flavoring works with this method of cooking the flank steak.

• If you don't have access to a grill, broil the steaks in the oven or use a stove top grill. I prefer the stove-top grill that cooks one side at a time for this recipe rather than an electric double-sided grill. I find it develops a crispier crust than the two-sided grill.

• You don't have to roll and cut the meat into pinwheels. You can leave the steak stretched out to cook, using the same time for medium rare. Slice into thin slices on the diagonal. These slices would be fabulous on sourdough bread with horseradish sauce.

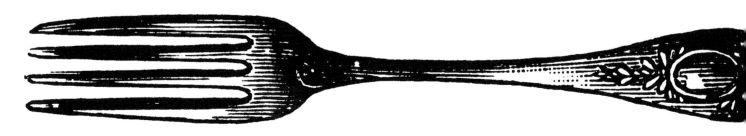

ENTRÉES

BEEF

• FRANKIE SEIVERS •

Summer Sausage

I see this recipe and think boys. For some reason, guys like to gnaw on manly chunks of meat. This makes a lot of tasty manly meat. It tastes just like the kind you buy in the store, only it doesn't have as much fat. A snack for the team after school? Paired with cheese and crackers for a team picnic? Tailgate nosh for the fans? Wonderful Christmas presents? Something for the guys to take back to college?

5 pounds ground chuck (80% lean or better)

5 heaping teaspoons Morton's Instant Tenderizing Salt (salt cure)

2 tablespoons liquid smoke

1 tablespoon mustard seeds

1 tablespoon garlic salt

1 tablespoon crushed red pepper

1. Mix all ingredients thoroughly and store in an air-tight plastic container. Store in refrigerator for 4 days, mixing each day.
2. On 4th day measure into 1 cup portions, shaping and firmly forming into desired shape. A long log works well.
3. Bake 150 degrees for 12-18 hours on broiling pan. Turn once.

Makes 11 rolls

Notes

• *Morton's Tenderizing Salt may not be at every grocery store you try. It comes in a blue, soft-sided bag and is used for home curing. Do not substitute regular table salt.*

• *This is a big old batch of meat. When I am mixing it during the four days of curing, I like to tear it into little chunks, about the size of a meatball, mix the different chunks up and then knead it all back together into one big ball.*

• *My oven will only go down to 200 degrees, but I cook the logs at that temperature for about 15 hours. Be sure to turn the logs when you still have about 3-4 hours of cooking left; the side that was touching the pan doesn't brown. The underside needs a few hours after it is flipped to lose its uncooked color.*

• *These freeze well; make a batch and have them on hand.*

• *Christmas gift? Great teamed with homemade preserves, flavored vinegar, a grand chunk of cheese, or a loaf of bread. Or check out the Cream Cheese Braids in the dessert chapter for the ultimate gift pairing.*

PORK

• SHIRLEY JARVIS •

Sunday Night Dinner
(Easy Pork Tenderloin)

This is what Sunday dinner is all about – slow-cooked roast meat swimming in delicious gravy. Use that gravy on hot mashed potatoes and add a salad for a memorable and easy meal. This one is good for everyone: little kids, football teams, parents, family gatherings.

5-6 pounds fresh pork tenderloin (unseasoned)

1 teaspoon hot sauce

$^1/_2$ envelope dry onion soup mix

1 can Healthy Request Cream of Mushroom Soup, undiluted

$^1/_2$ to $^2/_3$ cup red cooking wine

1. Trim the pork of all fat; rub with hot sauce and place in a large crock pot.
2. Sprinkle with the onion soup mix.
3. Mix the soup and wine together and spoon over the roast.
4. Cook for around 8 hours on low setting.
5. Remove meat from the gravy and let it stand for about 10 minutes before thinly slicing. Serve the gravy with mashed potatoes.

Serves 8

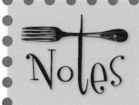

Notes

You could make your life even easier with the addition of a few vegetables to the crock pot: carrots, onions, potatoes. But leaving the meat all by itself produces a nice, clean flavor that blends well with side dishes. Your choice.

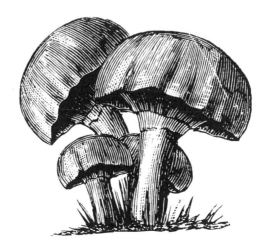

CHICKEN

•LEN POUSSON •

Chicken Paella

(Predecessor to Jambalaya)

My cousin, Len, has a houseful of active kids. She is an inspired Louisiana cook and knows how to fix food that kids love. This recipe is one of her favorites for feeding a crowd. It would be great at a tailgate. Flavorful without being spicy-hot, it has a little of everything in it: rice, three meats, black-eyed peas and tomatoes. The black-eyed peas add a slight sweetness that can be counter-balanced with an extra dash of hot sauce. Don't be intimidated by the long list of ingredients – it goes together pretty quickly once the meat is cooked. This would also work as a pre-game meal.

3 – 4 chicken breasts, cut into bite-sized pieces

$^1/_2$ cup olive oil

1 large onion, diced

2 -3 stalks celery, diced

1 red bell pepper, diced

1 green bell pepper, diced

4-5 cloves garlic, minced

$^1/_2$ cup green onions, sliced

1 package sliced mushrooms

1 cup ham or bacon

$^1/_2$ pound Kielbasa-style sausage, cooked and sliced

1 can black-eyed peas (optional)

1 cup diced tomatoes

3 cups long grain rice, washed and drained

4 cups chicken stock

1 teaspoon thyme

1 teaspoon basil

1 teaspoon saffron, (optional)

Salt and cracked black pepper to taste

Louisiana hot sauce to taste

1. Cut chicken into bite-sized pieces and season. In a 4 quart pot, heat olive oil over medium - high heat. Sauté chicken, a few pieces at a time, until brown on all sides. Remove and keep warm.
2. In same oil, sauté the onion, celery, garlic, green onions, mushrooms, ham or bacon, and sausage for 3-5 minutes until vegetables are wilted. Stir in the tomatoes and black-eyed peas, being careful not to mash the peas.
3. Add the rice and stir into vegetables. Cook gently for 3 minutes.
4. Stir in chicken stock and herbs. Season with salt, pepper, and hot sauce. Bring to a low boil and cook for 3 minutes, stirring occasionally.
5. Blend in chicken, then reduce heat to low and cover pot. Cook 30-45 minutes, stirring at 15 minute intervals.

Serves 8-10

Notes

• *This makes a really large batch of paella. Make sure the pot you use has enough room to accommodate the expansion of 3 cups of rice.*
• *You can use roasted chicken from the deli as a time-saver. If you have some chicken meat left over from making a chicken stock, you could use that.*
• *Turkey sausage works well in this dish.*

ENTRÉES

CHICKEN

• CATHY MELLOT •

CHICKEN Pot Pie

This is a signature dish for Cathy, and it is requested and anticipated at church and community events in her hometown of New Enterprise, Pennsylvania. Rich and full-bodied, it would be called Chicken 'n Dumplings in the south, but the starch is known as "pot-pie noodles" in her neck of the woods. This is a crowd-filling pleaser: big chunks of chicken floating in a flavorful sauce thickened by dumplings and vegetables.

$3^1/_2$ - 4-pound chicken or chicken parts

1 cup celery, chopped

1 medium onion, chopped

2 quarts water plus more

$1^1/_2$ teaspoons parsley

Salt and pepper to taste

2 tablespoons chicken soup base

5-6 potatoes, cooked and sliced

For pot pie noodles:

2 large eggs

4 cups flour

$^1/_2$ cup milk, as needed

1. Combine the chicken, celery, onion, water, salt, pepper and parsley in a large stock pot. Bring to a boil and skim off any foam that forms. Reduce the heat and simmer until the chicken is tender, at least 45 minutes, but longer is OK; you'll have a richer tasting broth.
2. Strain the mixture through a large sieve and return the strained broth to the stove. Spread the chicken out on a platter to cool. While the chicken is cooling, prepare the dough noodles.
3. When cool enough to handle, remove all the skin, cartilage and bones from the chicken. Tear the meat into bite-sized pieces. Set aside.
4. Bring the strained broth back to a boil, adding the chicken base and enough water to make $3^1/_2$ quarts (14 cups).
5. Drop the lightly floured dough squares into the boiling broth and cook until tender.
6. Add the cooked potatoes and prepared chicken; heat thoroughly. Serve in bowls.

For the dough noodles:
1. Beat the eggs and milk until light and frothy.
2. Gradually add the flour until a soft dough is formed. Handle the dough gently. It will shape up quickly – it should not be stiff or sticky.
3. Divide the dough into three equal pieces. On a floured cloth, roll each piece of dough out as thinly as possible. Cut into 1-inch squares. A pasta machine could be used for this step.
4. Flour the squares lightly and drop one at a time into the boiling broth.

Serves 8-10

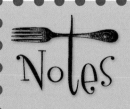

Notes

• *You could easily add vegetables to the mix if you wanted to up the health quotient. Peas and carrots are always good. Keep the size of the vegetables small and uniform for even cooking and appearance.*

• *If you just don't have the heart to face making dumplings from scratch, the cheater's method involves cutting refrigerated biscuit dough into small knots and dropping them in the hot broth.*

CHICKEN

• TILLIE LUNGARO •

CHICKEN Spaghetti for a Crowd

This is a quick and easy dish that feeds an army. You will need a wheelbarrow to get it to your event. It uses nearly every flavor of canned soup ever created, and combines it with chicken, tomatoes, cheese and pasta. Kids will eat it – and anyone else standing in the buffet line!

1 chicken, boiled, de-boned and chopped coarsely (chicken breasts can be used, but add 1-2 chicken bouillon cubes to the cooking broth to add the flavor the dark meat usually gives.)

1 large package and $^1/_2$ of small package of spaghetti, cooked al dente (see Perfect Pasta chapter for cooking tips for al dente)

1 can each:
  French onion soup
  cream of cushroom soup
  cream of chicken soup
  cream of celery soup
  cream of onion soup
1 pound cubed Velveeta cheese
2 10-ounce cans Rotel tomatoes, undrained
1 16-ounce can chopped tomatoes, undrained

1. Preheat the oven to 350. Prepare two large casserole pans with non-stick spray.
2. Combine the cooked pasta and chicken in an extra large mixing bowl.
3. In another bowl, combine all the soups, cheese and tomatoes.
4. Stir the sauce ingredients into the pasta mixture. You may want to do this in a couple of batches if the whole amount becomes unwieldy.
5. Divide mixture between prepared casseroles. Bake covered for 20-25 minutes.

Serves 12-15

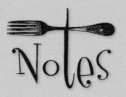

Notes

• *This makes a rich sauce that could easily be thinned with more spaghetti and extra chicken. The original recipe calls for 1$^1/_2$ packages of spaghetti, but I always go ahead and use two full packages, and there seems to be plenty of sauce.*
• *Substitute turkey-based Polish sausage that has been sliced and browned for the chicken. Or add it with the chicken.*
• *If you are in a hurry, use roasted chicken from the supermarket.*
• *A few veggies never hurt a casserole. Saute an onion and 2-3 stalks of chopped celery in a tablespoon of butter until softened. Add to the sauce mixture before combining with the pasta. These amounts are starting points – add more or less to taste. You could also throw in some mushrooms, sliced and sautéed in butter.*
• *The Rotel tomatoes add a little heat; substitute one large can of fire-roasted tomatoes if you prefer a quieter version.*
• *For a vegetarian variation, just leave out the meat – you still have a rich, delicious sauce full of protein. You might substitute some cheddar for half the Velveeta for a sharper cheese taste. I like using all cheddar or a mixture of cheddar and Monterey jack. You could even sprinkle on some Parmesan.*

CHICKEN

• FRANKIE SEIVERS •

CHICKEN spaghetti II

Wow – will this feed a crowd for not a lot of money! Rich and delicious, this is a simple-tasting dish of chicken and noodles in a creamy, cheesy sauce. Cooking the pasta in the broth really infuses it with the chicken flavor. Kids love it! Don't try to double this recipe; simply make it twice.

4 chicken breasts

2 quarts (8 cups) chicken broth

1 bell pepper, chopped

1 cup celery, chopped

1 cup onions (1 medium), chopped

1 pound spaghetti

2 cans cream of chicken soup

Salt and pepper to taste

³/₄ tablespoon Tiger seasoning

8 ounces cheddar cheese, shredded

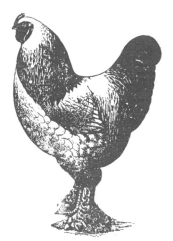

1. Preheat the oven to 400 degrees. Treat a 9x13-inch casserole with non-stick spray.
2. Boil and de-bone chicken breasts; cut into chunks. Reserve 8 cups of the cooking broth, which has been seasoned with salt to taste.
3. Bring the broth to a boil and add the pepper, celery and onion and chicken first, then add the pasta and cook until tender.
4. Add the 2 cans of soup to the mixture, season with salt and pepper to taste. Stir in the Tiger seasoning and mix well.
5. Add half the cheddar cheese and stir well. Pour the mixture into a 9x13 casserole pan. Top with the remaining cheese.
6. Bake for 40 minutes.

Serves 8 generously

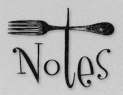

Notes

• *Tiger Seasoning is a blend of sodium, cornstarch and spices. If you can't find it, you could substitute a seasoning blend of your choice – almost any would work well with this dish. Think Cajun spice, Mediterranean or Greek, Italian blend – anything with a bit of spice and herbs.*
• *If you were in a big rush, you could use a roasted chicken from the supermarket and canned or boxed chicken stock.*

CHICKEN

• CAROL POWELL •

Church Chicken Casserole
For a Crowd

Carol prepares this frequently for church dinners and it always disappears. Do you have young children to feed? This is a great starting point casserole. Prepared as is, it tastes a lot like chicken and dumplings, but is much easier to fix. Children love its unassuming, comforting flavors. All sorts of things can be added to it, however, to make it spicier or more nutritionally complete, like vegetables or cheese. It can be made ahead or frozen. It feeds a crowd. It just may be perfect!

5 pounds chicken parts

$^1/_2$ cup sherry (or white wine)

1 medium onion, quartered

$^1/_2$ teaspoon curry powder

1 tablespoon salt

1 stalk celery

2 boxes long grain/wild rice

1 can cream of mushroom soup

1 cup sour cream

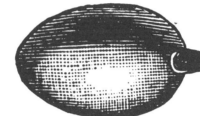
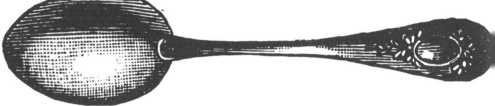

1. Preheat the oven to 350 degrees. Prepare a four-quart casserole or two, two-quart casseroles with non-stick spray.
2. In a large stockpot combine the chicken parts, sherry, onion, curry powder, salt, celery, and enough water to cover. Bring to a boil and skim off scum. Reduce heat and simmer until the chicken is tender – at least one hour, but longer will give you a richer broth. Add water to the pot as necessary.
3. Remove the chicken from the broth and cool; strain the broth and save.
4. Remove the skin and bone from the chicken and cut into bite-sized pieces. Set aside.
5. Cook the two boxes of rice according to package directions, substituting the saved broth for the cooking water.
6. Combine the soup and sour cream, mix well.
7. Mix all the ingredients – chicken, rice and soup mixture – and place in the casserole. Add a little more broth if you need to.
8. The casserole can be refrigerated at this point and held until needed, or frozen. When ready to serve, bake for 1 hour. If frozen, add 15 minutes cooking time.

10 servings

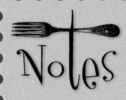

Notes

- *This casserole can go so many ways, it boggles the mind. Start with vegetables – try adding two cups of chopped, blanched broccoli and top with shredded cheddar cheese and a sprinkle of paprika.*
- *Mushrooms would be another good addition. Sauté them in a little butter before adding to the rice and chicken. You could throw a diced onion and a couple of cloves of minced garlic in the pan with the mushrooms.*
- *Other good veggie/cheese topper combinations include: asparagus/ Monterey jack; artichoke hearts/ parmesan; peas/ white cheddar.*
- *For some interesting texture, sprinkle the top with buttered breadcrumbs mixed into the cheese. Or try crushed potato chips – kids love the crunch.*
- *Want to go healthy? Use low fat sour cream and low sodium soup.*

CHICKEN

• FRANKIE SEIVERS •

Frankie's Fried Chicken

This comes from Frankie Seivers, who has been fixing this recipe a long time – first for her children (one of whom is University of Tennessee Football Hall of Famer Larry Seivers), and now for her grandchildren. It is a fixture at family gatherings, not just asked for but expected, along with her sugar cookies. Frankie says she isn't a fancy cook, she just fixes good old country food. She may not be a fancy cook, but she is a fabulous cook, and her food never fails to please. Her contributions are always highly anticipated at any potluck event. She says the secret to this recipe is the Kentucky Kernel Seasoned Flour. Look up comfort food in the dictionary and you'll find a picture of this fried chicken.

3 eggs
$^1/_2$ cup water
1 chicken, cut into pieces, skin on
Kentucky Kernel Seasoned Flour
Vegetable oil for frying

1. Heat at least two inches of oil in a large skillet or electric skillet until it reaches 350-400 degrees.
2. Mix the egg and water. Dip the chicken in the mixture and then dredge in the seasoned flour.
3. Fry in the pre-heated grease, skin side down, until golden on one side, about 30 minutes. Turn and cook on the other side. Drain on paper towels.

Serves 4

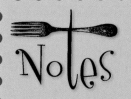

Notes

• Be careful about putting too much chicken in the oil too quickly. You don't want to lower the temperature of the oil and you don't want to crowd the pieces.
• Going healthy? This chicken can be baked instead of fried. You can even use skinless chicken. But – and this is a big but – dip the chicken in a little melted butter instead of the eggs before covering with flour. You might even want to spray the floured chicken pieces with some non-stick spray after they are placed on the baking sheet to keep them from drying out. Bake in a 375 degree oven for 20-40 minutes, depending on the size of the pieces and whether there is a bone involved. This is a great way to prepare chicken fingers.

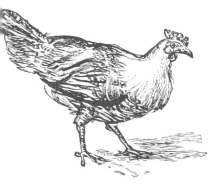
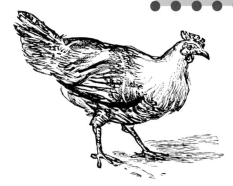
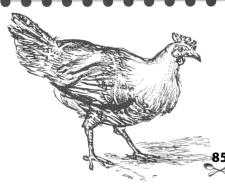

CHICKEN

• PAM MULLINS •

Hot Chicken Salad

I have one word for this dish: Mmm. The chicken shares the pan with fresh vegetables, cheese and almonds, but the piece de resistance are the potato chips on top. This is a one-way ticket back to the Fifties! This was served at a church affair (now THERE'S an oxymoron), and I watched the men in the crowd go back again and again for another helping of this casserole. Even young kids like it, but if someone has a mayonnaise phobia, they better not stop here. This makes a divine ladies' lunch with a fruit salad and sinful dessert. It also is at home on the buffet table at church or school.

2 cups cooked chicken, cubed

1 bell pepper, chopped

1 cup celery, diced

5 tablespoons onion, grated

2 tablespoons fresh lemon juice

1 cup mayonnaise (Hellmann's preferred)

1 cup potato chips, crushed

$^1/_2$ cup cheddar cheese, grated

$^1/_4$ cup slivered almonds, toasted

Parsley, finely chopped

Paprika

Salt and white pepper to taste

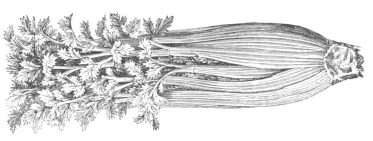

1. Heat the oven to 450 degrees. Place oven rack in the center of the oven. Prepare a casserole with non-stick spray.
2. Combine the chicken, vegetables, lemon juice and mayonnaise. Correct the seasoning.
3. Pour mixture into the prepared casserole and top with chips, then cheese, then almonds. Sprinkle with parsley and paprika for a colorful finish and bake for 20 minutes. Serve warm.

Serves 6

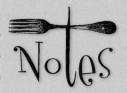

Notes

• *This is a mild, rich dish that looks better without big black pepper flakes floating around. Use the milder white pepper or eliminate the heat entirely.*

• *Since there is a lot of sodium in the chips and cheese, you won't need much added salt in this dish. Try salting your chicken lightly before adding it to the mixture – that will probably be more than enough for the whole dish.*

• *To toast the almonds: put nuts in a heavy skillet on medium high heat. Watch them closely – they are thin and will burn in a heartbeat. Toss and stir until they color slightly. Remove the pan from the heat immediately, stirring all the while, and pour into a bowl until ready to use. Take the time for this extra step – the flavor is significantly improved.*

• *Don't skip the parsley and paprika – both add color and flavor to the dish.*

• *You can make this dish healthier – if you must – by using low fat mayonnaise (Hellmann's makes a good one), baked potato chips and reduced fat cheese. Check your seasonings when you switch to low-fat. You may need a touch more salt and pepper to replace the lost flavor from the fat. I would pre-test the low fat version before serving it to a crowd to make sure you like it. I prefer a smaller portion of the real-deal version because the flavor and texture are so different.*

Baked Hot Wings

This is an easy recipe to modify; you can make the wings as hot or as mild as you like. Great finger food for kids in the milder version. Teens love them while watching a game on TV. The secret of these wings is that they are baked rather than fried – you can eat a lot more! Figure a generous $^1/_2$ pound of wings per adult serving, and then add a little extra for the pot. This recipe uses $2^1/_2$ pounds for a serving for four. If serving as an appetizer, figure about 4 wings per person.

$2^1/_2$ pounds wings

**Pre-mixed Cajun seasoning powder
(Tony Cachere and Paul Prudhomme are two favorites)
or Seasoning mix (recipe follows)**

Salt to taste (if it is not included in the seasoning powder)

Hot sauce (optional and highly recommended)

Dipping sauces: Ranch, Blue cheese

1. Pre-heat the oven to 400 degrees. Treat a shallow pan or cookie sheet with non-stick spray. Do not use a pan with high sides; the wings will not get as crisp. If you are making more than one pan in the oven at a time, switch pans to the top shelf during cooking. Otherwise the wings in the bottom pan won't get as crisp.
2. Spread the wings out in a single layer in the pan. Season heavily (or to taste) with seasoning powder.
3. Cook in the pre-heated oven about 15-20 minutes and then turn the wings over and season the other side. Cook another 15-20 minutes, or until crispy and tender.
4. Towards the end of this second cooking, you can sprinkle the wings with some hot sauce for a more traditional wing flavor.
5. Serve hot with dipping sauce, a large bowl for bones and lots of paper towels. And a few Tums.

4 servings

SEASONING MIX

2 teaspoons salt

2 teaspoons paprika

1 teaspoon cayenne pepper

1 teaspoon onion powder

1 teaspoon garlic powder

$^1/_2$ teaspoon cumin powder

$^1/_4$ teaspoon white pepper

Mix all the ingredients in a small bowl.
Combine thoroughly and sprinkle on wings.

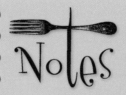

Notes

• *Play with your seasonings, adjusting the mildness to taste. I like to add a sprinkle of chipotle powder on top of the Cajun seasoning – it adds a smoky depth to the flavor. Smoked paprika is another interesting addition. No need to measure – just sprinkle on after the wings are laid out in the pan.*

• *Play with the hot sauce, too! There are lots of options out there: green Tabasco and chipotle Tabasco to name just two. I like to fix two pans of wings and flavor them each a little differently. This gives me an excellent excuse to eat more in the name of comparison.*

• *Don't limit yourself to Cajun spices for these. Try Chinese, Thai or Mexican mixes as well. Have fun on the spice aisle. You will need to change your dipping sauce when you change your spices – or just eliminate it all together – it just slows you down!*

• *Try bottled salad dressings for a quick and easy dipping sauce. Chunky blue cheese dressing is perfect for the traditional wings. If you are going Asian, try a spicy ginger sesame dressing. A creamy herb dressing with some fresh cilantro and a squirt of fresh lime juice added is perfect for a Mexican twist.*

• *Another dressing option is hot sauce added to some melted butter. Use about 8 tablespoons hot sauce per stick of butter for a nice, sinus-clearing hit of heat.*

CHICKEN

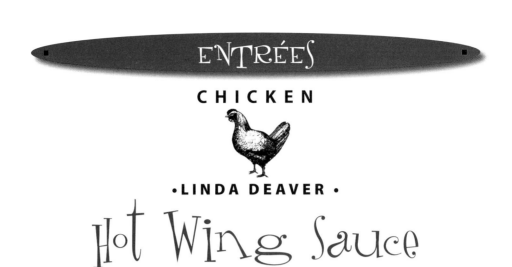

· LINDA DEAVER ·

Hot Wing Sauce

This flavorful recipe grills instead of fries the wings, and the hot sauce has an added element of sweet and sour that makes it different from traditional wing sauces. It will dress 8 pounds of wings. It is a great favorite with teenage males.

2 cups Frank's Red Hot Sauce
2 cups brown sugar
2 tablespoons red wine vinegar
1 stick ($^1/_2$ cup) butter

1. Combine ingredients and warm on the stove or in microwave.
2. Put wings in a zipper bag with the sauce and marinate two hours, turning bags several times.
3. Grill the wings on low, keeping a close watch, since the sugar in the sauce will burn easily. Cook about an hour, basting with sauce during cooking.

Serves 10 normal people or 6 hungry boys

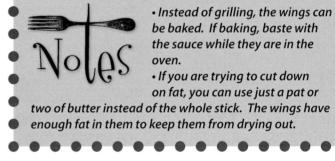

Notes

- *Instead of grilling, the wings can be baked. If baking, baste with the sauce while they are in the oven.*
- *If you are trying to cut down on fat, you can use just a pat or two of butter instead of the whole stick. The wings have enough fat in them to keep them from drying out.*

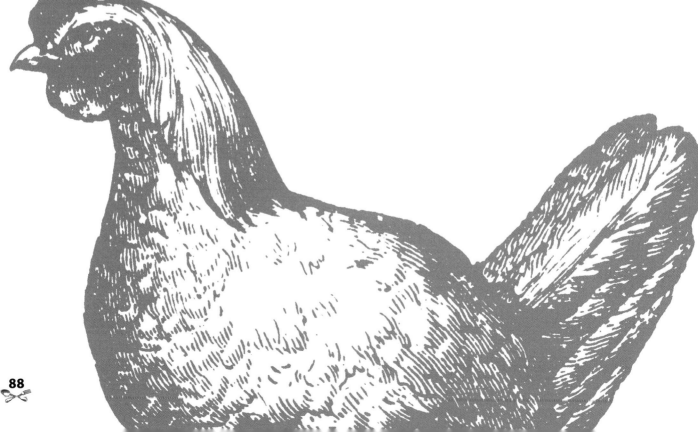

CHICKEN

• LEAH MOIR •

King Ranch Casserole

Yes, this casserole has been around for ages. When you've got a good horse, ride it! Chicken, cheese, and tortillas are layered in a flavorful sauce, sort of like a Mexican lasagna. Recipes like this are pure gold: simple, tasty, and inexpensive. It isn't too spicy for kids in spite of the chiles, which actually are quite mild. It is easy to gussy up with flavorful additions. This can headline a Mexican menu with sides of black beans and guacamole. Or slip it in the potluck line – it's a nice change from pasta and rice dishes.

1 whole chicken, boiled, skin removed and de-boned (see Notes)

1 dozen corn tortillas

1 small onion, finely chopped

1 package cheddar cheese (grated)

SAUCE

1 can cream of mushroom soup

1 can cream of chicken soup

1 small can of green chiles or fresh roasted (diced)

1 can chicken broth or fresh broth from cooked chicken (1 cup)

1. Preheat the oven to 325 degrees. Spray a large, oblong casserole with non-stick spray.
2. For the sauce: combine soups and chicken broth in a saucepan. Add green chiles. Stir until smooth and cook on low heat for about 10 minutes.
3. In the casserole dish, place a layer of 6 tortillas, torn into bite-sized pieces. Follow with half the pieces of cooked chicken, half of chopped onions, half of sauce, then grated cheese. Repeat layers ending with cheese.
4. Bake for 1 hour, uncovered.

Serves 6-8

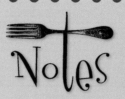 Notes

• *See the Master recipes for directions for cooking chicken in broth.*
• *You can substitute chopped pickled jalapenos for the chiles, or add them along with the chiles. Use ¹/₄ - ¹/₂ cup chopped jalapenos, depending on how hot you like it.*
• *Try adding a layer of salsa or enchilada sauce over the chicken for a flavor boost (my favorite modification). There are terrific jarred sauces and salsas in a variety of flavors available. Frontera makes a great one. Spread a generous ¹/₂ cup on top of the last layer of chicken before following with onions, sauce and cheese. Or stir it into the sauce.*
• *Add a teaspoon of chipotle chili powder to the sauce ingredients for a spicy, smoky taste (my other favorite addition).*
• *If you don't have tortillas, you can use restaurant-style white or yellow tortilla chips instead. Just don't crush them too finely; only smush them down enough to lay flat in the casserole.*
• *Garnish the cooked casserole with a sprinkle of loosely chopped fresh cilantro. Maybe finish with a squirt of fresh lime juice? It brightens the flavors.*
• *I have cooked this, covered, in a 275 degree oven for about six hours when I wanted it to be ready when I got home from work. I finished it in a 350 degree oven for about 10 minutes, uncovered, to dry it out.*

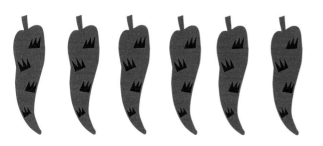

CHICKEN

• WEBB FRIDAY NIGHT FEASTS •

Chicken & Dressing Casserole

This is the recipe that has been used by every cook everywhere. It combines the classic flavors of chicken and dressing, moistened with creamy soups thinned with broth and optional sour cream. The stuffing absorbs all the chicken flavor and retains a wonderful moistness. It is the centerpiece for an easy "Thanksgiving Lunch" menu during the holidays; it is included every year at the football feedings since it is one of the most popular recipes with the kids. It is a great company dish, since you prepare it ahead of time and let it sit overnight before baking. This recipe doubles easily.

Note: this recipe must be refrigerated overnight before baking

4 large chicken breasts
Water, garlic, bay leaf,
1 can cream of chicken soup
1 can cream of mushroom soup
1 cup sour cream (optional)
1 package Pepperidge Farm stuffing
$^1/_2$ cup (1 stick) butter, melted

1. Prepare a roasting pan with non-stick spray.
2. Cook chicken breasts in a large pot of water flavored with a bay leaf, clove of garlic, and a stick of celery. Bring to a boil, skim off foam and lower to simmer. Cook 30 minutes (but longer is OK). Cool and chop coarsely, reserving 4 cups of broth. This can be done 2-3 days ahead.
3. Combine cream of chicken soup with $1^1/_2$ cups reserved chicken broth. Set aside. If using the sour cream, combine the soup with $^1/_2$ cup sour cream and one cup broth.
4. Combine mushroom soup with remaining $1^1/_2$ cups reserved broth. Repeat the quantities above if using the sour cream: $^1/_2$ cup sour cream, 1 cup broth.
5. Combine the melted butter and stuffing; mix well and fluff with a fork. Reserve $^1/_4$ cup for topping.
6. Spoon half of remaining stuffing in a greased baking dish. Top with half the chicken and half the chicken soup mixture. Repeat layers of stuffing, chicken and soup.
7. Pour mushroom soup over the layers; sprinkle with reserved stuffing mixture.
8. Cover and refrigerate overnight.
9. Pre-heat the oven to 350 degrees. Remove the casserole from refrigerator 15 minutes before putting into the oven. Bake covered for 30 minutes; uncover and continue cooking 15-20 minutes longer. Check for moistness and add broth if the casserole is drying out.

8 servings

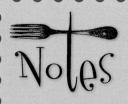

Notes

• *Shallow pans will bake for the shorter time*
• *For a stronger "Thanksgiving" taste, add 1 teaspoon poultry seasoning to the chicken soup mixture.*
• *A whole chicken can be substituted for the chicken breasts. The dark meat will add flavor and moisture. If using a whole chicken, prepare in the same way as with the breasts, and cook at least 45 minutes (see Master Recipes for detailed instructions for boiling a whole chicken.) Strain broth and meat and spread the chicken out on a large platter to cool. When cool enough to touch, remove bones, skin and cartilage; tear meat into bite-sized pieces.*
• *Serve with canned cranberries for a quick side, or choose one of the cranberry salads from the salad chapter.*

SEAFOOD

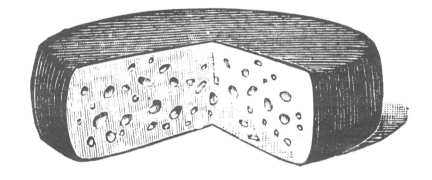

• LESLIE GALLAHER •

CRAB STRATA

Leslie has been tailgating with this recipe for years. It is a great company dish since it can be prepared ahead and must sit overnight. The egg-soaked bread puffs up during baking, making a wonderful surrounding for the savory rich crab and cheese filling. Pair it with fruit salad and garlic bread for an elegant meal. The seafood in this recipe makes it a little sophisticated for the kiddies; save it for a teacher's luncheon or tailgate, where adult palates can appreciate its flavor.

1 loaf French bread

2 small cans crabmeat (drained) or 1 pound frozen crabmeat or one 12-ounce package imitation crab meat, chopped

$^1/_2$ cup chopped celery

$^1/_2$ cup chopped onion

$^1/_2$ cup shredded Swiss cheese

$^1/_2$ cup shredded cheddar cheese

$^1/_2$ cup mayonnaise

4 beaten eggs

3 cups milk

$^1/_2$ teaspoon prepared mustard

Salt and pepper to taste

Dash cayenne pepper or hot sauce

1. Butter a 9x13-inch casserole dish.
2. Tear French bread into bite-sized pieces and scatter in the bottom of the casserole.
3. Layer crab over bread, then sprinkle on the celery, onion and cheeses, distributing evenly.
4. Blend together the mayonnaise, eggs, milk, mustard, salt, pepper and hot sauce. Pour over the bread mixture and refrigerate overnight.
5. Preheat oven to 325 degrees. Remove the casserole from refrigeration while the oven heats. Bake the casserole, covered, for 45 minutes. Uncover and bake an additional 15-20 minutes.

Serves 10-12

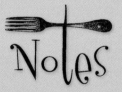

Notes

• *This dish could be modified easily to a kid-friendly, budget-conscious dish by substituting one pound of cooked chicken for the crab.*
• *Use a firm textured bread in this recipe. It even helps if the bread is a little stale; it will soak up more of the liquid without becoming too soggy. Regular sliced bread should not be substituted.*

91

S E A F O O D

BEST BARBECUED SHRIMP

This wonderful recipe was inspired years ago by the cooking of Paul Prudhomme. He mixes all his seasonings together before adding them, and he isn't afraid of using a lot of heat. This recipe, one of my family's favorites, creates the most wonderful sauce for dipping. We could actually do without the shrimp and just dunk bread in the fiery butter sauce. I like using a lot of herbs, both for their wonderful, fresh flavor, and to offset the heat of the pepper.

Seasoning mix:

$1/2$ - 1 teaspoon ground red pepper
   (cayenne works the best)

1 teaspoon white pepper

$1/2$ teaspoon salt

1 teaspoon thyme

2 teaspoons rosemary leaves

1 teaspoon oregano

1 pound large shrimp (unpeeled), rinsed and patted dry

1 stick ($1/2$ cup) unsalted butter

$1^1/2$ teaspoons minced fresh garlic

1 teaspoon Worcestershire sauce

$1/2$ cup bottled clam juice

$1/4$ cup beer, room temperature

1. In a small bowl, combine the seasoning mix.
2. Use a large skillet so the shrimp have room to move around. Heat the pan over medium high heat and add the butter, garlic, Worcestershire sauce. Stir in the seasoning mix once the butter is melted.
3. Add the shrimp to the seasoned butter and cook for 2 minutes, shaking the pan (versus stirring) to move the shrimp around.
4. Add the clam juice and the beer. Shake the pan and cook for about 2 minutes, until the shrimp turn pink. Remove from the heat.
5. Serve immediately with lots of French bread and napkins. And Tums.

Serves 4

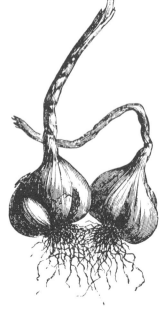

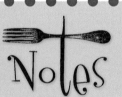

Notes

• *If you don't have beer, splash in some white wine instead. Oops! I spilled a little extra.*
• *I ration the cayenne pepper depending on who I am feeding. If you know your crowd loves hot, go for the full amount – and you could even add a sprinkle of red pepper flakes for a nice dash of red in the sauce. For a less adventuresome crowd, cut the pepper in half.*
• *If you happened to have some fish stock or shrimp stock in the freezer, you could use this instead of the clam juice. Save the shells from this go-round, boil them up and freeze the stock for the next time you fix the recipe.*
• *If you are serving more than four, make separate batches so all the shrimp have a chance to lay flat in the sauce and absorb flavor while they cook.*

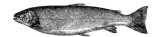
SEAFOOD

•SHIRLEY JARVIS•
FIERY CAJUN SHRIMP

This easy-to-prepare dish is full of flavor: herbs, garlicky butter and heat. There are lots of variations of this floating around, but this one is easy since it is baked in the oven. You can adjust the sauce ingredients according to the amount of shrimp you are using and the amount of heat you want. Serve with crusty French bread for dipping and lots of napkins for dripping – or maybe just a few rolls of paper towels.

5-6 pounds extra large raw shrimp in their shells

4 lemons, 2 juiced and 2 sliced thinly

2 sticks of melted butter

$^1/_2$ cup canola oil

$^1/_2$ cup Worcestershire sauce

4 tablespoons ground black pepper (or to taste)

1 teaspoon ground or crushed rosemary

2 teaspoons Tabasco sauce

2 teaspoon salt

3-4 cloves of garlic, minced

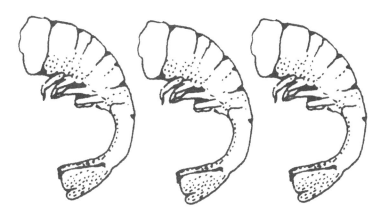

1. Preheat the oven to 400 degrees.
2. Rinse the shrimp in cold water. The little "legs" can be removed, if desired.
3. Layer the shrimp and lemon slices in a large pan.
4. Combine the remaining ingredients and pour over the shrimp.
5. Bake, stirring once or twice for about 15-20 minutes until cooked through.
6. Serve with crusty hot bread for dipping.

Serves 6-8

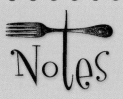
Notes
• *Because the shrimp are cooked with their shells on, the meat will not absorb too much of the sauce. The flavor and heat is in the sauce in which the peeled shrimp can be dipped for more intensity.*
• *Don't think you are doing your guests a favor by shelling the shrimp before cooking. Part of the fun is peeling them and getting messy. Plus, the sauce would annihilate peeled shrimp – it is designed to have enough flavor to penetrate the shells.*
• *This is good to serve in the summer on the patio while you are grilling. Just cover your table with spread-out newspapers and let everyone peel their shrimp right on the table. You will need a bowl for the sauce and dipping, though.*

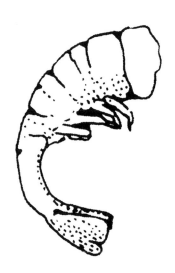

RECIPES

SOUPS AND SANDWICHES

SOUP

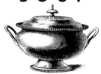

SANDWICHES

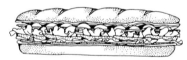

SOUP

chicken Gumbo

There are dozens of recipes for gumbo, but for it to be "authentic" Cajun it needs to have a roux (flour browned in fat and used as a thickener) and okra, also used as a thickener. Gumbo is a poor man's feast: the roux is an inexpensive way to add flavor to a lot of water and any animal caught in a trap. Long, slow cooking tenderizes any cut of meat. I've had gumbo made with rabbit, alligator, and duck, as well as seafood and chicken. It's all good! Gumbo can be spicy or not, but it always is flavorful, no matter what the heat level. Gumbo is best made ahead and left in the refrigerator a day or two for the flavors to marry – but if you are impatient and want a same-day meal, start it early in the day. This is a recipe that takes effort, but it feeds a grateful crowd.

STOCK:

1 whole chicken

3 quarts (12 cups) of water

1 onion, unpeeled

1 rib celery

1 bay leaf

3 cloves garlic, unpeeled

Salt to taste

SEASONING:

$1^1/_2$ tablespoons salt

1 teaspoon sweet paprika

$1^1/_2$ teaspoons white pepper

1 teaspoon red pepper

$^3/_4$ teaspoon black pepper

1 teaspoon garlic powder

1 teaspoon onion powder

$^3/_4$ teaspoon dry mustard

1 teaspoon cumin

1 teaspoon dried oregano

ROUX:

$^1/_2$ cup flour

$^1/_2$ cup fat (vegetable oil or solid shortening – not butter)

2 cups onions, chopped

2 cups green bell pepper, chopped

$1^1/_2$ cups celery, chopped

4 cloves garlic, minced

1 – 2 bags frozen okra (depending on your preference)

$^1/_2$ cup chopped onion (optional)

$^1/_2$ cup chopped celery (optional)

White rice

Filé powder (optional)

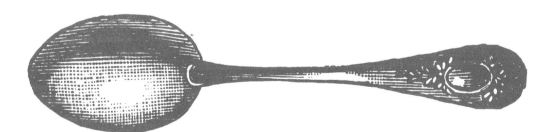

1. To prepare chicken and stock (this may be done several days in advance): put the chicken in a large stock pot with 3 quarts cold water, the onion, celery, garlic and bay leaf. Bring to a boil and skim off foam. Simmer for 1 – $1^1/_2$ hours, until the chicken falls from the bone, adding more water as the stock cooks down. Remove the chicken from the broth, spread out on a large platter to cool. Strain broth through sieve and return to stock pot. Remove the skin, bones and cartilage from the cooked chicken and tear the meat into bite-sized pieces with your hands. Set aside or refrigerate until ready to use.

2. Combine all the ingredients for the seasoning in a small bowl and mix well.

3. For the roux: In a large, heavy skillet (cast iron is ideal) heat the fat over medium high heat. Carefully add the flour so you don't splash the hot grease, stirring constantly. Turn the heat down to medium. Add just a little more flour if the roux seems wet; there should be no fat floating on the top of the mixture. It will be loose at first, but it thickens as it cooks. Stirring constantly, brown the roux until it is a deep brown, the color of milk chocolate. The texture is like a thin cake

continued on page 96

icing when you first start, but it gradually thickens as it cooks to something like chocolate mashed potatoes. Be patient; this is going to take a while. As the roux darkens, it cooks faster, so don't leave the pan alone for a minute. As the roux approaches the proper color, it will be changing color very quickly. Stir a lot! If it seems to be cooking too fast, just pull the skillet off the heat for a minute, continuing to stir. If it gets too dark, throw it out and start over. There is no way to salvage a burned roux.

4. The roux can be refrigerated at this point if desired. It will keep for a week in the fridge. Otherwise, add the chopped onion, celery, peppers and garlic to the warm roux and stir vigorously. It will look like very thick, lumpy cake batter at this point. Stir in two teaspoons of the seasoning mix; blend well. Pull the roux mixture off the heat.

5. Put the large pot of stock on medium high heat. Add enough water to the reserved stock to make 12 cups. If you must add a lot of water, throw in a bouillon cube for flavor, or use canned broth instead of water. Bring the stock to a gentle boil. Lower a large ladleful of hot roux into the stock and stir well until it is absorbed. Continue adding the roux a spoonful at a time to the stock until it is all incorporated. Let the mixture cook for about a half hour on low heat, skimming off any fat that floats to the surface. Try to avoid removing any floating vegetable pieces.

6. Sprinkle 2 teaspoons of the seasoning on the reserved chicken pieces.

7. After the gumbo has cooked down a bit and no more fat from the roux is floating to the surface (about $^1/_2$ hour), add the chicken and 1-2 teaspoons of the seasoning mix. Simmer uncovered for at least 2 hours, adding water or broth if it cooks down too much. Taste several times during the cooking time and add more seasoning mix as desired. Be cautious about using the entire amount – you will have a firecracker of a gumbo if you do. Adjust the salt to taste.

8. About $^1/_2$ hour before serving, bring the temperature up on the gumbo until it reaches a very gentle boil. If desired, add $^1/_2$ cup each of raw chopped onions and celery at this point. This will give you both very soft and firmer veggies in your gumbo. Simmer for about 15 minutes, and then add the okra. Cook until just tender and still bright green.

9. Serve the gumbo over hot white rice with some gumbo file (ground sassafras leaves) on the side for sprinkling.

6-8 generous servings

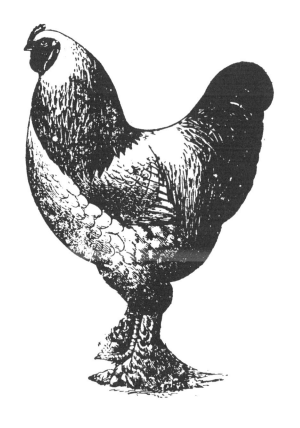

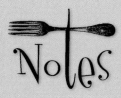

Notes

• The gumbo improves in the fridge overnight. Fix it a day or two before you need it.
• Don't store the gumbo and rice together. The rice will soak up all the moisture and leave you with a very dry gumbo. Add the rice at the last moment.
• Gumbo freezes beautifully. You can add more okra to it when you thaw and reheat it.
•Some people don't like the okra and leave it out, but the okra is a traditional gumbo ingredient used as a thickener.
• Gumbo filé, which is ground sassafras leaves, is also used as a thickener; it has a very strong flavor. Start with a sparing sprinkle on top of your gumbo and gradually add more to taste.
• A popular addition to chicken gumbo is polish sausage, sliced thickly. I like to brown the slices before I add them to the gumbo about halfway through the cooking time. They tend to get a little mushy if added too soon.
• If you want more flavor and less heat, cut back on the cayenne and black pepper in the seasoning mix. This is a very spicy mix and is too much for most children. If you wish, separate some gumbo and add just a little seasoning mix for the more timid palates in the group. The key is to taste as you go and stir well after every addition.
•This is a basic recipe that works well for most meats and seafood.

S O U P

• HELEN WALKER •

Shrimp Gumbo

This is a streamlined version of classic gumbo with a secret ingredient: brewed coffee. It comes from the heart of Cajun country and a wonderful cook, my aunt Helen in Lake Charles. She takes advantage of the convenience of Kary's Roux in a jar, which makes an authentic-tasting gumbo without the fuss (and if she uses it, it must be OK!). See the ingredients chapter for sources. This gumbo, with its distinct seafood flavors, is best suited to adult palates. Skip this one for the kids.

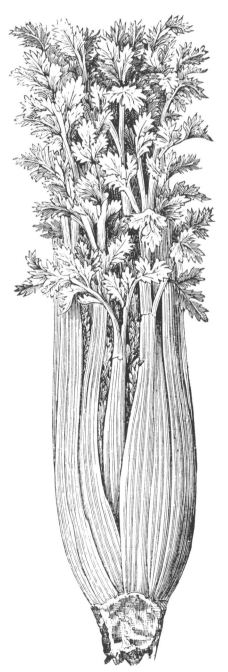

1 gallon (16 cups) water

1 14-ounce can chicken broth

1 10-ounce can Rotel tomatoes

$^1/_2$ cup brewed coffee

1 jar Kary's Roux (drain off the oil at the top of the jar)

1 cup chopped celery

1 cup chopped onion

1 cup chopped bell pepper

1 6-ounce can crab meat

Salt, black pepper, garlic powder to taste

2 pounds shrimp, peeled and deveined

1 16-ounce bag of frozen okra

Chopped green onion and parsley for garnish

White rice

1. In an 8 quart pot, combine the broth, Rotel tomatoes, coffee, and water to equal one gallon. Heat to a boil.
2. Add the roux a spoonful at a time, stirring after each addition until completely dissolved.
3. Reduce the heat to medium low and add celery, onion, bell pepper, and crab meat. Season to taste with salt, pepper and garlic powder. Cook until vegetables are tender, about 15 minutes. Skim excess oil as it floats to the surface.
4. Add the shrimp and bring gumbo to a boil; cook 8 to 10 minutes.
5. Turn off the heat and add the okra. Cover until ready to serve
6. Pour servings over cooked rice and top with onions and parsley.

Serves 10

SOUP

•RUBY HERRING•

Mother's Vegetable Soup

This vegetable soup is famous in our family. My mom always makes it whenever the extended family gets together. It is the perfect dish to hold on the stove until everyone arrives. We eat it for breakfast, lunch and dinner. It is always simmering on the stove, and someone is always eating it. It can be made ahead, frozen, reconstituted, added to – it just keeps getting better. Plus, it is good for you! This is easy to make, but it is time consuming. Start 1-2 days ahead. Take it to a sick friend. Prepare yourself; this recipe uses loose, indefinite or "to taste" quantities quite a bit. Read all the way through it before preparing it to map out how far ahead you want to start and which ingredients you want to include.

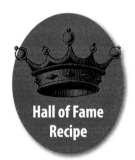

Hall of Fame Recipe

3-5 pound Chuck Roast

Olive oil

2 6-ounce cans tomato paste

1 large can peeled whole or cut up tomatoes

2 cloves garlic

1 onion, chopped

One small jalapeno pepper left whole with a sliver through body (optional)

Hot sauce to taste

1 small bag of mixed beans, pre-soaked, or several cans of mixed beans: pintos, kidney, northern, black

2 medium white potatoes, peeled and cut into irregular chunks

Additional onion (1 medium, chopped) and garlic (several cloves, chopped) (optional)

Italian Seasoning mix

Salt (start with at least 1 teaspoon) and pepper

1 small cabbage (more or less, depending on taste)

Assorted fresh and frozen vegetables: zucchini, squash, celery, green beans, carrots, peppers

$^1/_2$ cup fresh parsley, chopped (plus more for garnish)

$^1/_4$ cup Parmesan (plus more for garnish)

1. One or two days before serving, start the soup. A pressure cooker is best for this first step, but a large stock pot would also work. Brown the chuck roast in a little oil in the bottom of the cooker until deep brown. Add the two cans tomato paste, tomatoes – broken into pieces with your hands or an immersion blender, garlic, onion, and hot pepper, if using. Add enough water to cover, filling the cooker to the highest fill line. If using a stock pot, cover the ingredients with (at least) 10-12 cups water. Cook according to pressure cooker instructions until the roast is tender. In the stock pot, bring the water to a boil, then reduce the heat and cook gently until the meat is done and the water is flavorful, about an hour (but more is OK). Remove meat to a covered dish until cool enough to slice.

2. Remove all the fat from cooled meat while slicing. Cut into squares, like stew meat. Reserve in a tightly covered container with some of the broth from soup pot. Refrigerate until the serving day. The remaining broth can also be refrigerated until you are ready to assemble on serving day. It should be rich enough to add as much water as you need for the number you wish to serve. The meat and broth could also be frozen at this point. The broth should be refrigerated at least overnight to give the flavor time to develop. If you are in a hurry, you can skip this step, but only if you must.

3. Soak the bag of beans overnight. After they have soaked, rinse the beans several times before adding them to the soup.

4. The next day, heat the broth in a large stock pot. Add the pre-soaked beans which have been drained, and the potatoes. Bring to a boil and then simmer until the potatoes and beans are soft. The beans will need to cook at least an hour. If using canned beans, do not add them at this point;

continued on page 99

continued from page 98

they will become mushy. You can add extra chopped onion and garlic at this point, if you wish. (Do! Their flavor will be different from the garlic and onion you used in the original stock mixture.)

5. Begin to check your soup for seasoning. You will need to add a good bit of salt if you are making a large quantity. Taste for heat and add some pepper or a few shakes of hot sauce if the jalapeno needs supplementing. As your soup cooks down, you will add more water or other liquid. It is imperative that you keep checking for seasoning during the cooking process. A tablespoon of Italian seasoning mix can be added at this point. If you don't want to use a mix, add some dried herbs like oregano and basil. Start with a teaspoon of each.

6. After the soup simmers and the beans and potatoes soften, rest the soup overnight. It can be frozen at this point. If you don't have time to rest the soup again, go ahead and finish on the same day.

7. To finish the soup (day of serving): Warm the soup mixture on medium low heat. Cut up fresh vegetables into bite-sized pieces. Slice the cabbage as for slaw. How many veggies you add depends on how "soupy" you like your soup. Fewer veggies produce a wetter soup. Add frozen mixed vegetables, if using. Bring the mixture to a slow boil and boil for about 2 minutes. Turn the heat down to low medium. Add the prepared meat. Taste for seasoning.

8. Finish by adding the parsley and parmesan cheese. Turn the soup off and let it rest for about $1/2$ hour before serving.

9. Reheat very slowly and serve with some chopped parsley and parmesan in bowls for sprinkling on top. The soup can be left on a low simmer all day long. Turn off at night and be sure to add water if it cooks down too much. The completed soup can be frozen.

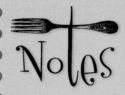

Notes

• This recipe is perfect for using all those various liquids you have in the fridge and freezer. Instead of plain water, use stock, either canned or prepared. If you save the water in which you boil veggies – throw it in. Any leftover gravy? Add it! A dash of wine? Yum. The one liquid you do NOT want to use is the water in which you soaked your beans – you throw away some of the gassy effect of beans when you toss out the soaking water. In fact, after soaking, rinse your beans several times and drain before adding to the soup for maximum no-gas benefit.

• Add as you go. As the soup gets eaten, throw in more veggies or meat or liquid. A can of tomatoes with their liquid is always a good addition when things get low. Always bring to a boil for a minute or two after a big addition and then lower the heat.

• I love adding tiny pasta to this soup – like orzo or the little alphabet pasta (kids love this, too!) Don't add big noodles unless you want a very thick soup with more solids than liquid.

• If you have added a lot of water, throw in some bouillon cubes or granules to amp the flavor back up. Be careful when salting, though, because these flavorings already have a good bit of sodium.

• Although you can add other meats - Italian sausage, chicken, duck, and pork – I like the pure combination of beef, tomatoes and veggies. The other meats can change the soup's personality significantly.

• The beauty of this soup is that you can tailor it to your own preferences. Low carb? Leave out the potatoes and noodles (but keep the beans for their fiber). Hate cabbage? Gone. Scared of veggies? Just use the meat, tomatoes, a little onion and garlic, and some of the small pasta (although vegetables cooked in this soup lose their distinctively veggie taste and sort of soak up the meaty-tomato-y flavor. This soup is a good way to get kids to eat new vegetables.)

• If you buy parmesan cheese in a big hunk, throw in a chunk of the rind that you might otherwise throw away. It adds fabulous flavor and you can either fish it out or avoid it when ladling up the soup. I know this sounds bizarre, but try it. The flavor addition is a revelation.

• Don't forgo the parsley as a garnish. Its fresh, green flavor is the perfect counterpoint to the slow-cooked flavors of the soup.

• Use a slow cooker to keep the soup going and free up a burner on the stove.

• Freeze single serving sizes for a quick lunch or dinner.

SOUP

•LEAH MOIR•

Turkey Minestrone Soup

This is quick, easy – and healthy. It goes together quickly, but it can be made ahead and left to simmer and mature. The frozen pasta with vegetables is a big time-saver. Good for a pre-game meal or swim-meet. Serve with cheese biscuits and a fruit salad.

1 pound ground turkey

Olive oil (optional)

1 quart low sodium chicken broth

1 package frozen garlic pasta with vegetables

1 15$^{1}/_{2}$-ounce can kidney beans, drained

1 14$^{1}/_{2}$-ounce can Italian seasoned tomatoes

1 small can tomato paste

Seasonings to taste: salt, pepper, garlic powder

1. Spray a large pan with non-stick spray, or lightly cover the bottom of the pan with olive oil and heat. Brown the ground turkey, adding seasonings such as pepper, salt, garlic powder, to taste.
2. In a large pot combine broth, pasta with vegetables, beans, ground turkey, tomatoes, and tomato paste. Bring to a boil. Reduce heat and simmer for 5 minutes.

Serves 6

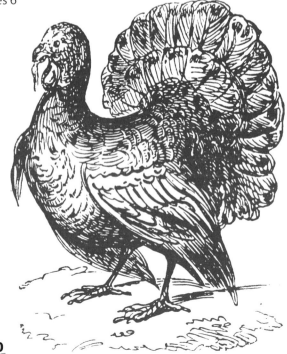

Notes

• *I know it is frustrating not to have exact seasoning measurements. But some of the ingredients, like the pasta, are pre-seasoned. Once you have combined the rest of the ingredients, start tasting and adjusting the heat and saltiness. All this tasting is the best part of cooking!*

• *If you want to heat things up a bit more, substitute a can of Rotel tomatoes for the seasoned Italian tomatoes.*

• *Although you can serve this soup immediately, I find that "resting" improves most soups. Bring the soup to a boil, then turn the heat to low and simmer for 15 minutes. Turn off the heat and let the soup rest for about 30 minutes (improvise on the time if you need to). Reheat slowly.*

• *Fresh herbs make a lovely addition to this soup. Try a handful of oregano, chives and/or rosemary. Add them toward the end of cooking so they don't turn bitter.*

• *You could change the meat – flavored chicken sausage would be good. Try the Italian variety, but lots of different flavors would work beautifully in this recipe.*

S O U P

•LEN POUSSON •

Quick Black Bean chili

This chili is quick and tasty, good on a cold day. It could be served over a baked potato, on top of a bed of corn chips, or on a hot dog from the concession stand. The black beans add wonderful fiber, and the lycopene in the cooked tomatoes is full of healthy benefits. If you used ground turkey instead of beef, you would have an easy, flavorful, low-fat meal the kids would love - especially if chips are involved.

2 pounds ground meat (beef or turkey)

1 onion, chopped

3 – 4 cloves garlic, minced

1 package chili seasoning

4 cans black beans (with juice)

1 can Rotel tomatoes (diced) or 2 cups chunky salsa

2 16-ounce cans tomato sauce or 1 28-ounce can

Salt to taste

Toppings:

Sour Cream

Corn Chips

Cheddar cheese

Red onions, chopped

Fresh cilantro, chopped

Fresh lime juice

1. Brown the ground meat in a skillet and remove to a paper towel to drain.
2. Add onions and garlic to the skillet. Cook until onions are wilted. If you used very lean ground beef, you may need to add a dash of olive oil to moisten the onion mixture.
3. Stir in the seasoning mix.
4. Smash 2 cans of black beans until thick, either with a potato masher or in a food processor. Just pulse, don't puree. You should have some chunks left in the mixture. Add the smashed beans and the other two cans of beans, along with the meat, tomatoes and tomato sauce to a stock pot.
5. Simmer for about 10 – 15 min. Taste for saltiness and correct seasoning. The package of seasoning already has salt, so be sure to taste before adding any more salt. Serve with your choice of toppings.

Serves 8

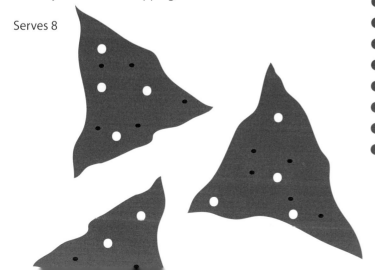

Notes

• You can substitute ground turkey or chicken for the beef for a low-fat variation. However, since there is much less fat in the poultry, be sure and spray the skillet with non-stick spray. Or use just a splash of healthy olive oil to keep things from getting too sticky. You also might need a little extra seasoning, since the meat is so bland. Try adding a little smoky chipotle chili powder – about a teaspoon should do it, although you may want to add gradually and taste as you go. If that is too assertive for you, try an extra shake or two of a mild chili powder.

• Try squeezing a little fresh lime juice on the chili right before serving for a wonderful taste brightener. It is amazing – and impractical if you are serving from a buffet. Keep a cut lime in your pocket for your bowl.

• You are dealing with a lot of tomato sauce here. The potential for stains is high. To get rid of tomato stains, try exposing them to direct sunlight. If that fails, rub some Lava soap in with a toothbrush and rinse under running water.

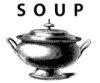

SOUP

•MISSY HUTTON•

Healthy Taco Soup

This is delicious on a cold day and has the familiar taste of tacos that kids love. A big variety of garnishes can really gussy it up. Plus, it has a lot of health benefits going for it: low fat, lots of fiber in the beans, and all the tomato-y lycopene. This goes together quickly, thanks to the taco and ranch dressing seasoning packets; it is hassle-free as it mellows in the crock pot. Serve with some guacamole, corn muffins and flan for dessert. It also is great on hot dogs – perfect for the concession stand.

1 pound lean ground beef, or stew meat cubes

1 onion, chopped fine

2 cloves garlic, minced

Olive oil

1 package Ranch dressing

1 package Taco seasoning

1 10-ounce can Rotel tomatoes

1 17-ounce can of corn, undrained

3 15-ounce cans of beans, undrained (pinto, black, kidney, northern, chili)

1 10-ounce can tomato sauce

2 cans (20 ounces) water or beef broth

Olives

Cheese

Sour Cream

Tortilla Chips

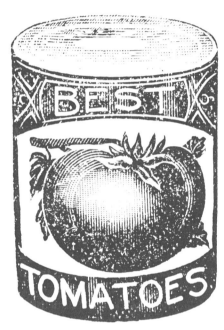

1. Pour a thin film of olive oil in a large skillet. Heat on medium high; when hot add the beef. After the beef begins to brown, add the chopped onion and garlic. Cook until the onions soften, around 5 minutes.
2. Sprinkle the ranch and taco seasonings on the meat mixture and continue cooking another few minutes until the seasonings soak in and flavor the meat.
3. Transfer the meat to a crock pot and add the Rotel tomatoes, corn, beans, tomato sauce and broth.
4. Set the crock pot on low and cook for 8-10 hours. When ready to serve, garnish with shredded cheese, chips, sour cream and olives.

Serves 8

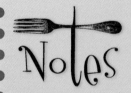

Notes

• Authentic chili uses beef cubes rather than ground beef; you get a bigger hit of beef flavor in each bite. But you can use ground beef or ground turkey if you prefer.
• Want some heat? Throw in a sprinkle of cayenne or chili powder. Garnish with chopped jalapenos.
• To keep the low-fat vibe going, you could use low-fat cheese, reduced fat sour cream, and baked tortilla chips.

Sandwiches

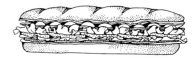

Brisket Sandwiches

These are perfect to send on the bus after a game. Or eat at a tailgate before the game (a little too rich for the athletes before the game, however.) Use the freshest bread you can get your hands on – I order mine from a bakery ahead of time, to be picked up the day of serving. One large brisket will make about 20-24 sandwiches.

Nana's Garlic Brisket, sliced (page 76)

Fresh sourdough bread, sliced

Creamy Horseradish sauce

Cheddar cheese slices (optional)

For each sandwich: spread horseradish sauce on both pieces of bread. Cover with meat, being sure to get some of the flavorful topping in each sandwich. Add cheese, if desired. Wrap each sandwich individually with plastic wrap for the freshest result if you are making ahead.

Serves 20-24

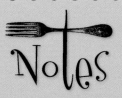

Notes

• *Experiment with bread and cheese: try a rye or pumpernickel, or a crusty Italian loaf. I like the sourdough best because it enhances rather than competes with the flavor of the brisket.*

• *Pepper jack or provolone cheese would be good, too. Try making a platter with a variety of bread/cheese combos: Italian bread and provolone; rye bread with Swiss cheese; pumpernickel and pepper jack.*

• *If you are serving the sandwiches on a platter, dampen a few paper towels with water and lay them gently on top of the pile of sandwiches. Cover the entire plate with plastic wrap or a dish towel until ready to serve.*

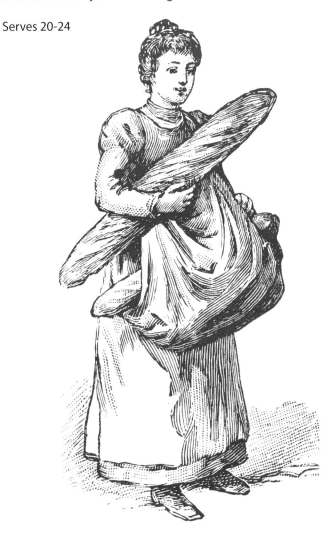

Sandwiches

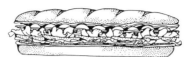

• PATTI PEARSON •

Ham Delights

Simple yet so good! These go together quickly. Kids love something they can eat with their hands, and adults love the classic combination of ham and cheese boosted with a little onion and mustard. Good for a tailgate or post-game feeding frenzy.

3 packs Pepperidge Farm party rolls (other brands may be used)

$^1/_2$ pound (2 sticks) butter

3 tablespoons prepared mustard

3 tablespoons poppy seeds

1 small onion, grated

1 teaspoon Worcestershire sauce

1 pound Virginia baked ham - shredded thin

$^1/_2$ pound baby Swiss cheese - sliced thin

1. Preheat the oven to 400 degrees.
2. Split rolls in half with a long bladed knife (leave rolls attached to each other).
3. Melt butter and add mustard, seeds, and onion. Spread mixture on both sides of rolls.
4. Layer the ham and cheese. Put rolls together and return to aluminum pan.
5. Now slice rolls into the individual rolls. Cover the pan with foil (you may freeze at this point) or proceed to heat. Heat 10 to 15 minutes until cheese begins to melt.

Serves 6-8

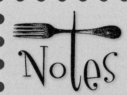

Notes

• *Try this with other meat and cheese combinations: turkey and pepper jack cheese; corned beef and Swiss; roast beef and cheddar.*
• *Prepare several combinations of meat and cheese and present each variety on a different platter. Serve with pickles and olives on the side.*

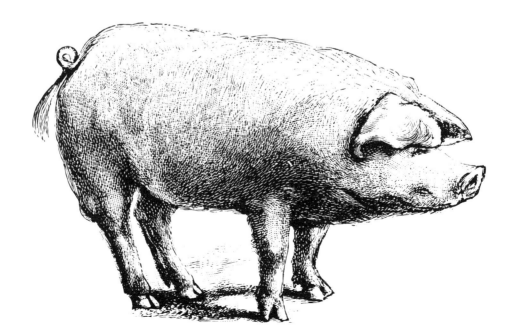

Sandwiches

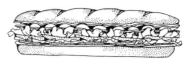

• DIANE ROBBINS •

Hot Chicken Salad Sandwiches

This is a lovely luncheon dish, easy to prepare and quite elegant. The crunch of the buttered bread is the perfect foil for the rich chicken salad topped with sauce. Children won't get too excited about this one, but their moms might. Serve with a fruit salad and light dessert.

16 slices of Pepperidge Farm bread, crusts trimmed and one side buttered

2-3 cups cooked chicken, chopped

3 hard-boiled eggs, chopped

4 ounces fresh mushrooms, chopped and cooked in 2 tablespoons butter

$1/4$ cup ripe olives, chopped

2 tablespoons onion, minced

Juice of $1/2$ lemon

$3/4$ cup Hellmann's mayonnaise

1 can cream of chicken soup

1 cup sour cream

2 tablespoons dry sherry (optional)

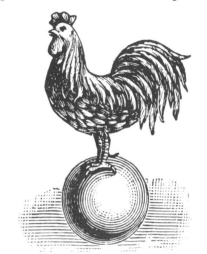

1. Preheat the oven to 325 degrees. Butter the bottom of a 9x13-inch casserole. Line with 8 slices of bread, butter side down.
2. Mix the chicken, eggs, cooked mushrooms, olives, onion, lemon juice and mayonnaise and taste for seasoning. Spread over the bread.
3. Top with the remaining pieces of bread, butter side up.
4. Mix together the soup, sour cream and sherry and pour over the bread. Bake for 30 minutes. If it looks like things are drying out too much, cover loosely with a piece of tinfoil, but don't close it down tight. You don't want to create condensation.

Serves 8

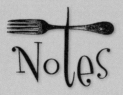

Notes

• *Instead of Pepperidge Farm, try nice, substantial bread from the bakery with a chewy crust. It holds up well to the hot salad and sauce, providing a nice, chewy texture.*

• *Use a flavorful mushroom like portabella. Cook fresh mushrooms in the hot butter until they lose their moisture and volume. Make sure you cook them until they "weep" out their moisture so your casserole won't be too wet. If you are in a hurry, you can use a jar of mushrooms, but the flavor won't compare.*

• *You can use lower fat versions of the sour cream and mayonnaise for a healthier recipe. When I am trying to be good, I lower the fat content on most of the ingredients, but leave one (or two?) full fat for their flavor and texture. It isn't quite as virtuous, but it helps the flavor of the final result.*

• *If you like a little oomph in your salad, add a sprinkle of white pepper or a shake of hot sauce. You don't need a lot, since this is not supposed to be a spicy dish; however, just a little adds that much-desired layer of flavor without the heat.*

Sandwiches

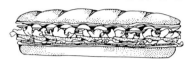

•LEAH MOIR•

Pizza Sandwiches

So this is like that frozen bread pizza that kids love. It is so easy to make: bread, cheese, pepperoni and a jar of tomato sauce. The trick is to hollow out the baguette a bit to make room for all the good stuff. These are easy to make assembly-line fashion. And pretty darn good. Best hot, they still hit the spot room temperature, which makes them a good choice for bus food.

1 French baguette about 20 inches long

Red pasta sauce

Pepperoni slices

Pre-shredded four-cheese Italian mix

Italian seasoning

Crushed red pepper (optional)

1. Preheat oven to 400 degrees.
2. Cut baguette into 4 sections and then slice in half horizontally.
3. Using your fingers, gently scoop out and discard some of the soft inner part of the bread, leaving a one inch thick shell.
4. Spread tomato sauce evenly among the bread shells, about 2 tablespoons per shell. Layer on the pepperoni and then cover generously with the cheese mix. Sprinkle each sandwich with Italian seasoning mix and crushed red pepper, if desired.
5. Place the sandwiches on a baking sheet and bake about 20 minutes, until the bread is nice and crispy. Serve immediately.

4 servings

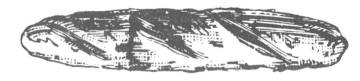

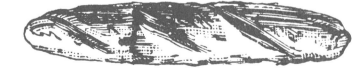

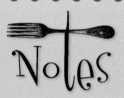

Notes

• *Slicing the bread in half makes a nice, crunchy crust. If you prefer a deep-dish pizza effect, slice off only the top third of each baguette section, scoop and stuff as usual. Use the top portion of bread in another recipe (it would make great bread crumbs.) You will have a higher ratio of bread to meat than when cutting the bread in half.*

• *I use turkey pepperoni and I am hard-pressed to notice a difference from the real thing in this recipe. I highly recommend it.*

• *You can use sausage instead of pepperoni – either Italian sausage or browned breakfast sausage. If you use Italian sausage, cut it into narrow slices and brown before using.*

• *You could vary your cheese, too, using a combination of provolone and mozzarella, and finishing with a sprinkle of Parmesan.*

• *This is, in fact, your basic hot meat 'n cheese sandwich. If you don't like the pizza twist, slap a little mustard and mayo on the bread, pile up some roast beef or turkey, cover with Monterey Jack or smoked Gouda and bake until gooey. The variations are endless.*

• *Get fancy and add a few veggies in the scoop-out after you lay down the red sauce and before you add the meat and cheese. Try diced onions, thinly sliced bell peppers, mushrooms, jalapenos.*

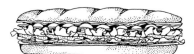
S a n d w i c h e s

• **PATTI PEARSON** •

Hot Dogs Deluxe

These are great on the buffet line since they are already "dressed" on the inside and no one has to slow down to add condiments. Kids love them because they are fun to eat; adults enjoy the sophistication of the tasty pastry. The puff pastry is a cinch to use - you won't have any unattached buns floating around with this recipe!

1 tablespoon butter

1 large onion, sliced

1 package frozen puff pastry sheets, thawed

$^1/_2$ cup spicy brown mustard

8 hot dogs

2 cups shredded cheddar cheese

1 pound bacon, cooked crisp and crumbled

8 servings

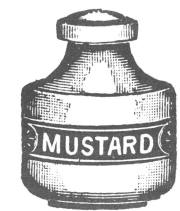

1. Take the frozen pastry sheets out of the freezer and begin thawing while you prepare the rest of the recipe. Preheat the oven to 400 degrees. Lightly grease a large baking sheet.
2. Sauté the onion in butter until tender. Set aside to cool.
3. Starting with the first pastry sheet, roll it into a 14x12-inch rectangle on a lightly floured surface. Cut the rectangle in half, and then cut each half into half again, to make four rectangles.
4. Brush each rectangle evenly with the mustard, leaving a $^1/_2$-inch border around the edges. Place a hot dog lengthwise onto half of each rectangle. Top evenly with the onion, cheese and bacon. Moisten the edges with water; roll up, jellyroll fashion. Press edges to seal.
5. Repeat with remaining sheet of pastry and hot dogs.
6. Place hot dogs, seam side down on baking sheet. Bake for 20-25 minutes, or until browned.

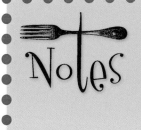

If hot dogs make you queasy, you could try ham instead and eliminate the bacon. Or maybe turkey and Monterey jack cheese. Any meat and cheese will taste good wrapped in puff pastry and heated in the oven. Get creative.

Serves 8

Sandwiches

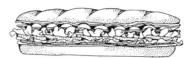

Meatball Sandwiches

Could there be an easier sandwich? The hard part is making the meatballs ahead of time. This makes a wonderful sandwich for the bus ride home after a game, or a tailgate party.

1 recipe Cheesy Meatballs (page 75)
1 jar marinara sauce
Provolone cheese, 8 thick slices
8 crusty rolls

1. Preheat the oven to 350 degrees.
2. Combine the meatballs with the jar of marinara sauce in a deep saucepan. Heat gently.
3. Slice each roll in half and scoop out a little of the tender filling of each piece. You are trying to make room for the meatballs so the sandwich will close nicely – otherwise the meatballs have a tendency to get away from you.
4. Layer in the cheese on the bottom half of the roll and top with enough meatballs to fill – 2-3, depending on the size of your meatballs.
5. Spoon extra sauce over the meatballs and cheese. Spread a little extra sauce on the top of the roll before closing up the sandwich. The inside should be moist, not sloppy, drippy wet. Repeat with all the rolls. Place on a flat baking sheet treated with non-stick spray.
6. Bake the rolls in the oven until the cheese is hot and gooey and the bread crisps up, about 10 minutes.
7. If using for a picnic, let the sandwiches cool and wrap individually in plastic wrap, then in tinfoil.

Serves 8

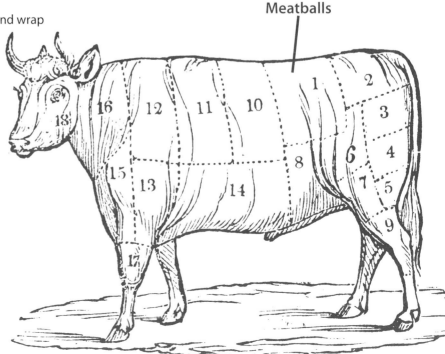

Meatballs

Sandwiches

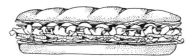

•CINDY BAIRD•

Mom's Pimento Cheese

This is a terrific recipe that never fails to please the kids; they love the mild, cheesy flavor of Velveeta. It can be halved easily. Use it to make sandwiches for the bus before or after a game. Pair pimento cheese sandwiches with fried chicken at a tailgate. It is the perfect, protein-rich after-school snack spread on whole wheat or sourdough bread. Or stuffed in some celery. Or try a dollop on a baked potato or hamburger patty.

2 pounds Velveeta cheese, grated

8 ounces cream cheese, grated

1 package cheddar cheese (Kraft in gold package)

1 large jar pimentos (drained)

1 teaspoon sugar

1 tablespoon grated onion

Garlic powder to taste

Pepper to taste

1 pint salad dressing (Kraft Miracle Whip preferred)

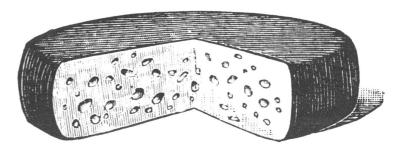

1. Combine all ingredients in a very large bowl. You may want to work in batches, since this makes a lot. This will make it easier to ensure you don't have any unblended pockets of ingredients. If using a food processor to blend, add the pimentos at the very end, or they will be pulverized and invisible.

Yield: 2$^1/_2$ quarts (10 cups)

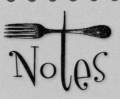

Notes

• *This makes a quite sweet, mild pimento cheese. If you want a tangier spread, leave out the sugar and use regular mayonnaise (I like Hellmann's) instead of Miracle Whip.*

• *If you want a sharper cheese taste, eliminate the Velveeta and use only sharp cheddar cheese, or use half Velveeta and half cheddar to preserve the easy spreading texture of the Velveeta.*

• *Try adding a splash of dill pickle juice to cut some of the richness. If you want to get crazy, throw in 4-5 chopped pickled jalapenos. It makes a flavorful yet not too hot spread. Or you could substitute some hot pepper jack cheese for a portion of the cheddar cheese.*

• *If raw onion gives you bad dreams, just leave it out. Try substituting Penzey's shallot-pepper spice (see ingredients chapter).*

• *Pop the Velveeta cheese and cream cheese in the freezer for about 15 minutes to make them easier to grate.*

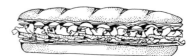

Sandwiches

• SHIRLEY JARVIS •

Cooked Pimento Cheese

This used to be cooked in a double boiler, but now a microwave does the trick. This produces a nice, homogenized finished product, slightly sweet but with a very subtle tang from the vinegar. Leave out the sugar to cut down on the sweetness. You would think that cooking would dramatically change the texture of the dish, but it doesn't. This is very spreadable, with a kid-friendly cheesy taste.

1 pound Velveeta

2 tablespoons milk

1 tablespoon sugar

$^1/_4$ cup white vinegar

3 large jars diced pimentos

$^1/_2$ cup mayonnaise

8 ounces finely shredded mild cheddar cheese

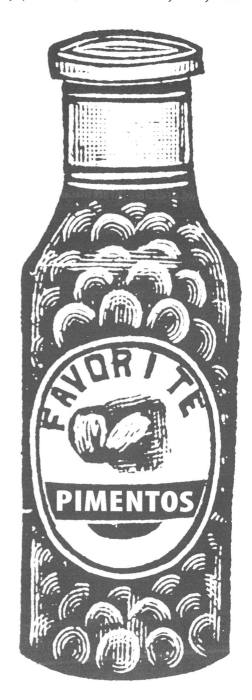

1. Spray the bottom and sides of a large microwaveable bowl with non-stick spray.
2. Melt the Velveeta with milk at 50% power at intervals of 2-3 minutes, stirring between intervals. Do not use full power – it will burn the cheese.
3. When the Velveeta is melted, add the sugar and vinegar; stir. Microwave again at 50% power for 1 minute.
4. Add the pimentos and microwave again at 50% power for 1 minute; stir.
5. Add the shredded cheddar, which will melt from the heat of the mixture without microwaving.
6. When cooled, stir in the mayonnaise. Add enough to reach desired consistency.

RECIPES

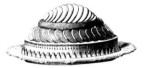

SIDE DISHES

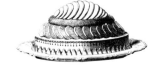

•RUBY HERRING•

Nana's Baked Beans

There is no excuse for serving undoctored baked beans unless you are sitting around a campfire and have to open the can with a little gadget on your key chain. Baked beans are always a favorite at any gathering since they compliment so many meat dishes and are pretty inexpensive. Boys love 'em for the obvious reason. It is so easy to make beans more flavorful – and the addition of salty (bacon?), sweet (molasses? brown sugar?), and savory (mustard? ketchup?) make this humble dish interesting and complex for the taste buds. Play with the ingredients; the open can is only a starting point.

4-6 strips of bacon, chopped into large pieces

1 medium onion, chopped finely

1 bell pepper, chopped finely

2 large cans Bush's spicy baked beans

2 tablespoons spicy brown mustard (or more to taste)

4 tablespoons ketchup

2 tablespoons brown sugar or molasses

Splash of balsamic vinegar

1. Preheat the oven to 375 degrees. Spray a large, shallow casserole dish with non-stick spray.
2. Sauté the bacon strips until some of the fat is rendered, but the bacon has not yet started to crisp. Remove to a paper towel. Leave the fat in the skillet.
3. Sauté the onions and peppers in the bacon fat, draining off some of the grease if the mixture is too wet (puddles of fat hanging around). Cook until the vegetables are soft. Remove to a paper towel to drain.
4. Dump the beans into a large bowl and add the vegetables and bacon. Add the mustard, ketchup, sugar and splash of vinegar and stir gently until well combined.
5. Pour beans into the pan and spread evenly. Cook uncovered for 45 minutes, or until the beans look thick and bubbly.

Serves 8-10

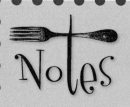

Notes

• *These amounts are not hard and fast. You can increase any of the individual ingredients to suit your taste.*
• *If you are rushed, you don't have to pre-cook the onions and peppers. Just chop into a small dice and add to the beans. Layer the uncooked bacon on the top so it can crisp as it cooks. And, as awful as it sounds, the bacon fat adds flavor to the beans, so you may not want to drain the partially cooked bacon, but just dump it in the bowl with the beans. Ditto the veggies cooked in the grease – forget draining them on the paper towel.*
• *Use a nice, spicy mustard – it adds so much character to the dish. If you have nothing else, of course add plain old "hot dog" mustard, but a flavored, grainy mustard is much better.*

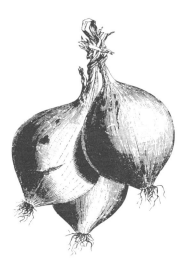

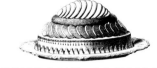

•SHIRLEY JARVIS•

Spicy Baked Beans

This is a fabulous recipe, made unusual by the addition of pineapple and sausage. It serves 12 easily, and can be halved for a smaller crowd. My family eats this until we fall unconscious.

4-5 (16-ounce) cans of Pork and Beans

1 large onion, chopped

1 green pepper, chopped

1 pound good pork sausage, browned and drained (I like the hot variety)

1 cup brown sugar (not packed)

1 cup Hunt's Spicy Honey barbecue sauce

dash of ketchup

2 tablespoons prepared mustard

2-4 tablespoons Worcestershire sauce

1 medium can crushed pineapple, undrained

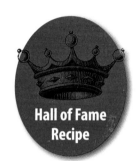

Hall of Fame Recipe

1. Preheat the oven to 350 degrees. Prepare a large casserole with non-stick spray.
2. Combine all ingredients in a very large bowl; mix well. Pour into prepared casserole.
3. Bake for 45 minutes.

Serves 12

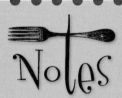

Notes

• To make this vegetarian, just eliminate the pork sausage and use meat-free canned beans.
• Try substituting some barbecue pork or beef for the sausage.
• You could also use bacon instead of sausage: lay uncooked chopped bacon strips across the top of the casserole, covering it completely, and bake.
• This makes a fairly juicy dish. I like to dry mine out a bit by giving it a finishing bake at 400 for about 15 minutes. It makes all that sweet spicy stuff nice and gooey.
• If you don't have a can of crushed pineapple, just toss a can of pineapple chunks in the processor, pulse a few times, and drain off about half the juice before adding to the dish.
• This makes a sweet dish – you could halve the sugar if you like beans with more bite.

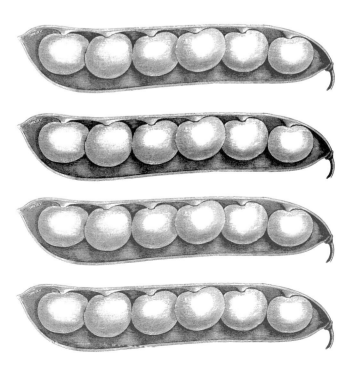

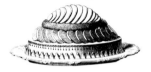

• WEBB FRIDAY NIGHT FEASTS •

Broccoli Casserole

Fast and easy, and the kids like it! This basic casserole has been a staple at the high school football dinners for years – and no wonder. It always gets eaten and it makes a good vegetarian option if you put lots of cheese on top. This doubles easily.

2 packages chopped, frozen broccoli
$^1/_2$ – 1 can cream of mushroom soup
$^1/_2$ cup mayonnaise
1 egg, lightly beaten
1 small onion, chopped
Salt and pepper to taste
Grated cheddar cheese
Pepperidge Farm cracker crumbs

1. Preheat the oven to 350 degrees. Treat a 9 x 13-inch casserole with non-stick spray.
2. Cook and drain broccoli.
3. Mix broccoli with soup, mayonnaise, egg, onion and seasonings and pour into the treated casserole dish.
4. Top with cheese and crackers. Bake 30 minutes.

Serves 6-8

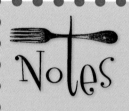

Notes

• *What? No exact measurements? You can figure you will need at least 1 cup of cheese to cover the ingredients, but you may prefer a thicker layer. Use all of the soup if you like a wetter dish.*
• *Don't wear yourself out steaming and chopping fresh broccoli. The frozen option captures most of the vitamins and is so much easier. Plus, by the time it gets jumbled with all the other ingredients and bakes, fresh is going to taste just like the frozen.*
• *Some people cannot abide mayonnaise. Substitute sour cream for the mayo and you still have a wonderful dish.*

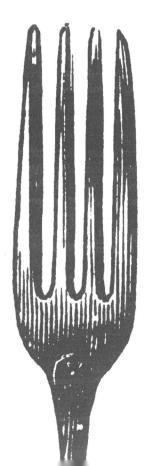

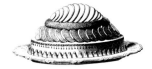

•PATTI PEARSON•
Cornbread Casserole

This is a rich dish that works well with soup, chili, or salad. It is more like an incredibly moist, cheesy corn bread. It is a good choice for vegetarians.

1 cup butter (2 sticks)
1 16-ounce can cream corn
1 16-ounce can whole kernel corn, drained
1 cup sour cream
1 package Jiffy corn muffin mix
2 teaspoons sugar
3 beaten eggs
One small package of pizza cheese or your choice of cheese

1. Preheat the oven to 325 degrees.
2. Melt butter in an extra large casserole dish (this recipe will bubble over and make a mess if your container isn't large enough).
3. Mix together the two corns, sour cream, muffin mix, sugar and eggs and pour in casserole dish.
4. Bake for 35 minutes.
5. Sprinkle cheese on top and return to oven just long enough for cheese to melt.

10 - 12 servings

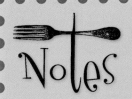

Notes

• *This recipe is good without the cheese.*
• *If you want to increase this recipe's fire power, try adding a tablespoon of chopped jalapenos (or a small can of chopped green chiles if your crowd is faint of heart) and top it with Pepper Jack cheese.*
• *Shredded cheddar is a tasty, colorful choice for a cheese variation or addition.*
• *A sprinkle of paprika on top of the cheese is a nice garnish.*

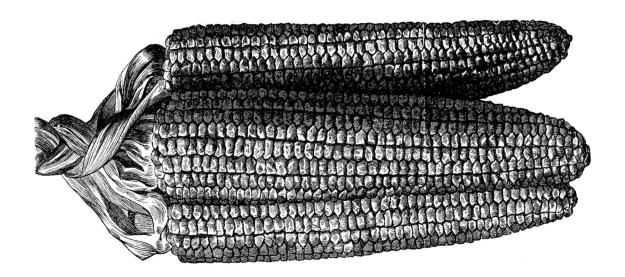

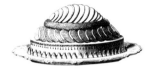

SIDE DISHES

•SHIRLEY JARVIS•

Corn Pudding

This is simply the best corn casserole I have ever had. It is a Shirley Jarvis family favorite and the perfect way to use fresh corn. It clearly is not diet food with two cups of whipping cream, but it is so worth the splurge! It has a rich, unadulterated corn taste – no onions, peppers or other vegetables – just sweet corn wrapped in a fluffy, buttery pudding. Try it just once and it will become one of your "go-to" recipes. Kids love it!

$^1/_4$ **cup sugar**

3 tablespoons flour

2 teaspoons baking powder

1 teaspoon salt

Pepper or hot sauce to taste

5 eggs, room temperature

2 cups whipping cream

$^1/_2$ **cup (1 stick) unsalted butter, melted**

6 cups fresh corn (or frozen)

1. Preheat the oven to 350 degrees. Grease a large casserole (at least four quarts.)
2. Combine the sugar, flour, baking powder, salt and pepper.
3. In a large bowl, beat the eggs until light and frothy. Add the whipping cream and melted butter.
4. Stir in the dry ingredients and the fresh corn. Pour into prepared casserole.
5. Bake for 45 minutes or until set. Cover with foil if the pudding begins to brown too much before setting.

Serves 6-8

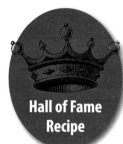

Hall of Fame Recipe

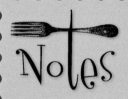

Notes

• *Don't use canned corn in this recipe; if fresh is unavailable, substitute frozen.*
• *I like to sift the dry ingredients into the wet ones to avoid any unincorporated lumps of baking powder.*
• *Although this recipe is perfect as it is, it modifies easily. When I didn't have the whipping cream, I made the recipe using half sour cream and half 2% milk. It was still divine.*
• *If you want a less sweet dish, cut the sugar in half.*
• *If you want to de-emphasize the sweet even more, use the pepper. I like to use white pepper in these lighter dishes.*
• *If you want to just blow it out of the water, add some chopped jalapenos – about 3 tablespoons, and sprinkle with shredded sharp cheddar cheese – at least 1 cup, but enough to cover the surface of your casserole generously. Don't add anything else, though. The beauty of this recipe is the intense simplicity of flavor.*
• *This recipe can be halved easily. Use 3 eggs for a firmer texture, 2 for a looser one. But go ahead and make the whole thing; I promise it will get eaten. And it freezes well after it is baked.*
• *To make this dish a little less overwhelming for the heart, you can use half and half instead of full cream, and cut the butter in half. I would not use a substitute for butter, however. The flavor would be compromised. If you want to be even more sensible, substitute 2% milk (not skim) for half of the cream called for.*

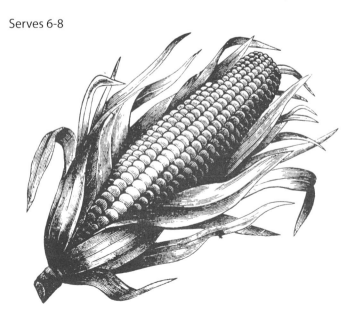

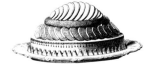

·PAM MULLINS·

Cream Corn Casserole

This is as old-fashioned and southern as it gets. It is similar to Tillie's Corn Casserole, but it doesn't have as many vegetables, and the onions are cooked in bacon grease, which changes the flavor in a big way. This is a rich, creamy casserole the kids will go for. This sits well at a buffet, but it won't last long.

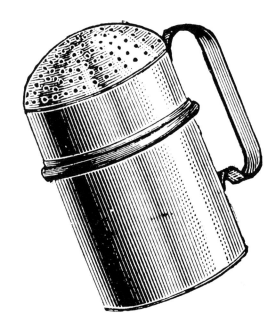

4 slices of bacon, fried crisp and crumbled

Grease from cooked bacon

1¹/₄ cups crushed cracker crumbs

1 onion, chopped fine

1 17-ounce can creamed corn (about 2 cups)

2 eggs, beaten

1 cup milk

1 cup grated cheddar cheese

4 ounces canned pimento, drained and chopped

Salt and pepper to taste

1. Preheat the oven to 350 degrees. Prepare a casserole dish with non-stick spray.
2. Mix ¹/₄ cup of the cracker crumbs with 2 tablespoons of bacon grease and and crumbled bacon. Set aside.
3. Cook onions in remaining bacon grease and combine with crumb mixture.
4. Combine the remaining crumbs, corn, eggs, milk, cheese and pimento. Season to taste with salt and pepper. Pour mixture into prepared casserole dish.
5. Top with crumb/bacon mixture. Bake uncovered for 45 minutes.

Serves 6

Notes

• *Don't substitute fresh corn in the recipe – although you could add some to the creamed corn. It will give you added texture – add about 1 cup.*

• *Corn and jalapenos just go together – add some if you want to play with your food. Chop about 2 tablespoons (or to taste) and throw them in.*

• *Use a variety of cheeses if you'd like – although cheddar is hard to beat.*

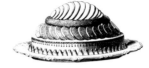

•HELEN WALKER•

Macque Choux (Smothered Corn)

This dish, pronounced "mock-a-shoe," is an old Cajun staple, one my mother's family grew up eating. A lot of recipes for this dish include cream and butter, and maybe even some crawfish. But this lighter, simpler version uses olive oil and the short-cut seasoning trick of salsa. This recipe does have visible vegetables in it other than the corn, so younger children may balk if they are vegetable-phobic. You could use a yellow bell pepper instead of the standard green ones to disguise its presence. Even though it is simple, the flavors of this dish are impressive and it is wonderful at a buffet, served hot or room temperature. It doubles or triples easily and can be made ahead and frozen.

2 tablespoons olive oil

1 medium onion, chopped

1 medium bell pepper, chopped

8 ears of fresh corn, shucked, cleaned with kernels sliced from the cob (4 cups)

1 Roma tomato, peeled and chopped

4 tablespoons of thick and chunky salsa

Salt, pepper and garlic powder to taste

1. Heat olive oil in a large pot. Add the onions and bell peppers and sauté for 5 minutes.
2. Add the fresh corn, salt, pepper and garlic powder. Stir fry on low heat for 15-20 minutes.
3. Add the Roma tomato and salsa. Cook another 10 minutes. Serve hot.

6-8 servings

Notes

• *If you are feeding a crowd, you may want to substitute frozen corn for fresh to save time.*
• *This is an easy recipe to add or subtract from. If you don't like the ratio of onions and/or peppers to the corn, add or subtract.*
• *If you like more kick in your corn, add of few dashes of hot sauce. You could also use one of the pre-mixed Cajun spices readily available on the spice aisle.*
• *Play with the salsa - try a smoky chipotle salsa, or maybe a really heated version. A salsa verde would be interesting, too.*

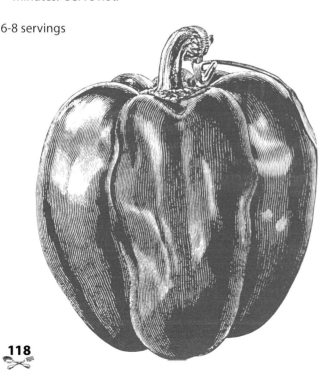

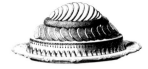

·TILLIE LUNGARO·

Tillie's Corn Casserole

This delicious recipe doubles easily and feeds a crowd. It comes to me from my Aunt Tillie in Lake Charles, Louisiana. She is active in a Mardi Gras Crewe there and knows how to throw the perfect party. Her recipes are always requested. This one is colorful and cheesy, full of chopped vegetables and a rich binding sauce. Young children love corn and this dish pleases all ages.

1 can cream style corn
1 can whole kernel corn
2 beaten eggs
1/4 cup crackers, crushed
1/4 cup evaporated milk
1/4 cup butter, thinly sliced or diced
1 cup carrots, finely chopped
1 small jar pimentos, drained
1/4 cup bell pepper, finely chopped
1 rib celery, finely chopped
1/4 cup onion, finely chopped
1 teaspoon sugar
1/2 teaspoon salt
12 drops Tabasco
1 cup cheddar cheese, shredded
Paprika for garnish

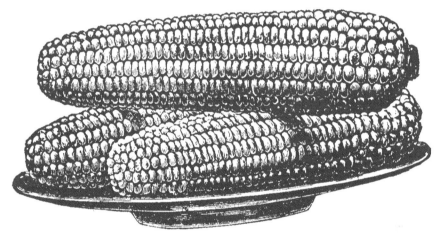

1. Preheat the oven to 350 degrees. Treat a large baking dish with non-stick spray.
2. Combine all ingredients and pour into a large casserole sprayed with non-stick spray.
3. Sprinkle with paprika and bake for 30 minutes.

Serves 8

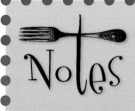

Notes

• *If you are fixing this for younger kids, chop the vegetables until they are no longer recognizable; they will still add their flavor and nutrition. Eliminate the pimentos, Tabasco and paprika – or at least cut down on the hot sauce. Taste as you go.*

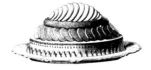

SIDE DISHES

• FRANKIE SEIVERS •

Old Fashioned Macaroni & Cheese

This recipe has been around forever – or at least ever since Velveeta has been produced. Frankie served this first to her kids, and now her grandkids love it too. It tastes like home. There are other, fancier recipes for this old favorite, but this one is perfect for feeding a lot of kids, no matter what their age. It is very mild and lightly cheesy, smooth and comforting.

1 large box (15-16 ounces) macaroni

1 stick ($^1/_2$ cup) butter

20-24 ounces Velveeta cheese cut into cubes

4 eggs

2 cups milk (more if mixture needs loosening)

Cheddar cheese, shredded

1. Preheat the oven to 350 degrees. Treat a 9x13-inch pan with non-stick spray.
2. Boil the macaroni in heavily salted water until al dente. Drain in a colander (for pasta cooking tips, see Perfect Pasta).
3. In the same pot melt the butter and the cheese cubes. Stir constantly until the cheese is melted; add the macaroni and stir until it is thoroughly coated with cheese mixture.
4. Beat the eggs and milk together and pour over the macaroni. Add a little milk if the mixture is too stiff.
5. Pour into the treated pan and top with cheddar cheese.
6. Bake 30-45 minutes or until set. Let the pan sit about 15 minutes before serving.

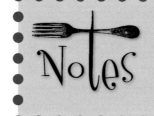

Notes

If you want a more sophisticated flavor, substitute sharp cheddar for some or all of the Velveeta – however, the presence of Velveeta ensures a smooth, melting texture.

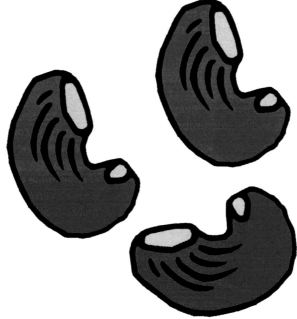

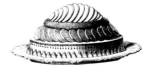

Overnight Company Potatoes

Instant potatoes?? Yes! When you goose them with cream cheese, butter, sour cream and cheddar cheese and then let them sit overnight before baking, they lose any "instant" identity. Just because it's easy, doesn't mean it isn't good! This is a great way to feed a crowd, and I highly recommend serving them with the brisket recipe.

5 cups instant mashed potatoes

4 cups warm water

2 cups milk, slightly warmed

8 ounces cream cheese, room temperature

One stick ($^1/_2$ cup) unsalted butter, melted

$^1/_2$ cup sour cream

Grated cheddar cheese (optional)

Garlic powder

Fresh chives, snipped

Salt and white pepper

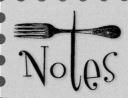

1. Mix potato flakes with warmed water and milk in an extra large bowl. You need plenty of room to stir all the ingredients without spilling.
2. Blend together the cream cheese, butter and sour cream. Add the mixture to the rehydrated potatoes.
3. Season with garlic, salt and white pepper (milder than black pepper and it looks prettier than black pepper in the potatoes.) Just keep tasting until you have it the way you want it. Start with at least 2 teaspoons of salt – this makes a lot of potatoes!
4. Turn into a large casserole that has been treated with non-stick spray. Sprinkle with chives and cheddar cheese, if using. Refrigerate overnight. (Do NOT skip this step – it eliminates the instant potato taste!)
5. Preheat the oven to 350 degrees.
6. Bring out of the refrigerator about 30 minutes before baking to bring the dish up to room temperature. Bake until heated through and the cheese is melted, around 30 minutes, maybe more, depending on your oven and how warm the potatoes were before baking.

8-10 large servings

Notes

• *To add a bigger garlic flavor than garlic powder gives, I like to smash 4-5 cloves of garlic and put them in a saucepan with the butter. Bring the butter to a boil, and then simmer a few minutes. Let the garlicky butter sit and cool for at least 15 minutes. Remove the garlic before adding the butter to the potatoes. This butter could be prepared in advance and refrigerated.*
• *If the potatoes need loosening, add more sour cream. If they are really thick, splash in a little more milk.*
• *I have used skim and 2% milk in this recipe, and it is fine. You could also use lower fat sour cream. If you use lower fat liquids, I would use a little extra cheddar cheese on top to replace the lost flavor.*
• *Sprinkle the top with some paprika for a colorful garnish.*

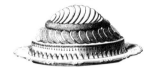

•RUBY HERRING•
FK Potatoes

These potatoes are named after their creator – or at least the fellow who introduced them to our family – Father Kemper. A dear friend of my family and clearly a brave soul, he accompanied us on a number of our vacation adventures. He fixed these potatoes for us once, and they became an instant family favorite. They are cousins to hash browns without the crispy crust. They have a wonderful savory finish from the paprika and onions that is excellent with roast meat, although the dish is hearty enough to serve with just a salad on the side for a light supper. The potatoes should cook for a while, so this is a great make-ahead dish. They improve overnight in the refrigerator.

Note: my mother never uses a recipe for these – she just adds ingredients until there are enough potatoes to serve however many show up for dinner. The amount of onion is always a bit less than the potatoes. She adds paprika until the potatoes are the right color – a lovely deep russet.

> **3 large potatoes, peeled and diced**
> **2 large onions, diced**
> **Olive oil (or canola oil, if preferred)**
> **Salt and pepper to taste**
> **Sweet paprika**

1. Heat a large skillet with high sides over medium high heat. Add enough olive oil to generously coat the bottom of the skillet.
2. When the oil is heated, add all the potatoes and onions at once and stir vigorously.
3. Begin seasoning with salt, pepper and paprika. Start with one tablespoon of paprika, a teaspoon of salt and $1/2$ teaspoon of pepper. Stir well to coat all the potatoes with seasoning. Add more paprika (its flavor makes this dish) until the potatoes reach a deep reddish-brown color. You want to get the potatoes to the right color with the paprika while they are still uncooked; stirring too much after they have tenderized will turn them to mush.
4. Once you like their color, cover the potatoes and onions and simmer on medium low until they are tender, at least thirty minutes. Begin tasting for salt and pepper and add more if necessary (they should already be the right color so you shouldn't need more paprika).
6. Gently stir the potatoes occasionally during their cooking time. Be careful not to stir too vigorously once the potatoes are tender; the texture will become too creamy. You want to have chunks of potatoes left, much like a potato salad.

4-6 servings

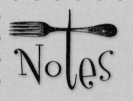

Notes

• *This is the blue-print for any quantity of FK potatoes you want to fix. Start by dicing potatoes until it looks like you have enough for the number of folks you want to feed. Three potatoes feed about 4-6. The amount of onion you add should be a bit less than potato – a 3/2 ratio of potato/onion is good. Increase the amount of paprika until the potatoes turn the right color. Season with salt and pepper to taste.*

• *You could add a layer of shredded cheddar cheese on top and pop under the boiler until the cheese melts. This would transform the dish into a wonderful entrée for vegetarians. A cup of cheese should give good coverage, unless you are using a really large-diameter pan. Shred enough cheese to create a solid layer over the top of the potatoes.*

• *For a marvelous flavor boost, try using smoked paprika. I would use half smoked, half sweet paprika in this dish. Too much of the smoked paprika could overpower the potato taste.*

• *This dish would be great heated up with spices – chipotle chili powder, or even chopped jalapenos (especially if you are going to add the cheddar cheese on top!). Start with a teaspoon of chili powder or a tablespoon of chopped jalapenos and add more to taste, of course.*

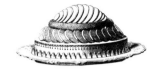

•TILLIE LUNGARO•

Hash Brown Casserole

OK, so you aren't going to lose weight eating this recipe. But I promise you won't care! This dish is a perennial favorite with any age, teeth or no teeth. Use it for breakfast or dinner. It is a revered potluck staple.

1 2-pound bag frozen hash browns

Salt and pepper to taste

1 onion, finely chopped

8 ounces sour cream

1 cup cheddar cheese, shredded

1 can cream of chicken soup

2 sticks (1 cup) butter

3 cups corn flakes, crushed

1. Preheat the oven to 300 degrees.
2. Spread potatoes in an 11x13 casserole sprayed with non-stick spray. Season to taste with salt and pepper.
3. Next, layer the chopped onions on top of the potatoes.
4. Melt one stick of butter and pour over vegetables.
5. Combine sour cream, cheese, and soup and heat in microwave for 45 seconds. Pour on top of the onions.
6. Melt last stick of butter and combine with corn flakes. Spread on top of casserole.
7. Bake for 1 hour.

Serves 6-8

Notes

• *This casserole can easily be spiced up. Add sliced jalapenos scattered over the onions.*
• *Try a sprinkle of chipotle chili powder over the potatoes and in the corn flake mixture for a smoky hit.*
• *Add crisp, crumbled bacon on top of the potato layer.*
• *After about 45 minutes in the oven, check the casserole to see if it is drying out. Cover loosely with tinfoil if you need to.*
• *You could easily cut down on the butter to save calories. Use only a few tablespoons poured over the vegetables, and only enough to moisten the corn flakes.*

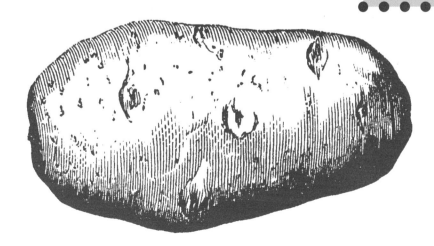

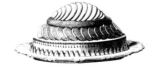

SIDE DISHES

·SHIRLEY JARVIS·

Hot German Potato Salad

This terrific recipe eschews mayonnaise altogether. Instead it uses oil and vinegar to dress the potatoes. The tart taste blends wonderfully with the salty bacon and the flavor of the potatoes is much more dominant. Try it with Reuben sandwiches on grilled rye bread.

6-8 slices of bacon, cooked crisp and crumbled very fine

3-4 pounds small red potatoes

2-3 tablespoons minced celery hearts

5-6 small green onions, sliced

$^1/_2$ cup vinegar

$^1/_2$ cup canola oil

$^1/_4$ cup water

Salt and pepper to taste

1. Wash and slice thin, unpeeled potatoes. Boil them slowly in salted water until just tender. They are done when the tip of a knife slides into them easily. Drain.
2. Add the onion, bacon and celery.
3. Combine the vinegar, oil, water, salt and pepper in a sauce pan. Bring the mixture to a rolling boil. Pour over the warm potatoes and stir carefully.
4. Serve warm. Leftovers can be microwaved to warm.

Serves 8

Notes

• *When the dressing and potatoes are both warm, the potatoes absorb more flavor.*
• *You could substitute a fruity olive oil for the canola oil. I have had this with apple cider vinegar, and it is a wonderful variation.*
• *This makes a tart salad. If you want something a little less piquant, reduce the amount of vinegar you use by $^1/_4$ cup.*
• *I like to add a little extra bacon.*
• *This makes a generous amount of dressing. You could start with half the amount and add more as your taste dictates. However, you need to be careful not to turn your potatoes to mush as you distribute the dressing carefully.*

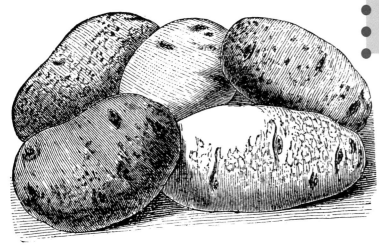

126

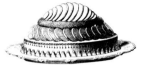

Roasted Potato Salad

This is an interesting take on potato salad. The roasted potatoes have a more robust flavor and different texture from boiled potatoes, and there isn't a boiled egg in sight. The dressing is a creamy vinaigrette enhanced with fresh parsley and chives. Younger kids rarely approach any potato salad with affection, but older kids will enjoy this, and the adults will love it.

3 pounds small red potatoes, cut in a large dice

2 onions, cut into fourths

6 cloves of garlic, minced

$^1/_4$ cup olive oil

$^1/_2$ cup mayonnaise

$^1/_2$ cup sour cream

$^1/_4$ cup fresh lemon juice

3 tablespoons chopped fresh chives

$^1/_4$ cup chopped fresh parsley

1 teaspoon salt

1 teaspoon white pepper

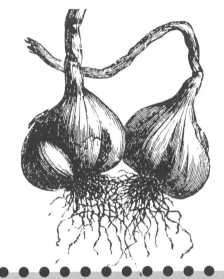

1. Preheat the oven to 400 degrees. Toss the potatoes, onions, and garlic with the olive oil and spread in a shallow-sided baking pan. Roast for 30-40 minutes, until the potatoes are tender and browned. Cool.
2. Combine the mayonnaise, sour cream, lemon juice, chives, parsley, salt and pepper in a large serving bowl. Mix well.
3. Add the potatoes and onion. Toss gently until the vegetables are well-coated. Cover and chill.

Serves 12

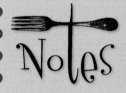

Notes

- *Try adding some crisp bacon crumbles and sprigs of fresh parsley for a garnish.*
- *You could add some blue cheese crumbles or Feta cheese for a heartier salad.*
- *Want a surprise? Add about $1^1/_2$ teaspoons of horseradish.*
- *Do not substitute dried herbs for fresh in this salad. Their flavor is too sharp. You need the lovely, green taste of the fresh herbs to contrast with the roasted vegetables.*

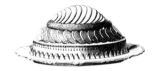

•SHIRLEY JARVIS•

Shirley's Potato Salad

This is a great basic, slightly sweet potato salad recipe made without boiled eggs. The curry and nutmeg add the "what is that?" element. This is especially good with ham and pork dishes.

4-5 pounds white or red potatoes

²/₃ cup finely diced celery hearts

²/₃ cup finely diced sweet onion

2 tablespoons sweet salad cubes with juice (sweet pickle relish)

1 teaspoon salt

1 teaspoon sugar

Canola oil

Pinch of curry powder

Pinch of nutmeg

²/₃ cup mayonnaise or a mixture of mayonnaise and sour cream

Paprika for garnish (optional)

1. Peel and dice the potatoes. Place in a pot of cold water and bring to a boil. Lower the heat and cook until tender, about 10-15 minutes.
2. DO NOT STIR, and drain potatoes thru a colander; sprinkle with the sugar and a bit of canola oil; set aside to cool.
3. Dice the onion and celery. Add the sweet salad cubes, mayonnaise, curry powder and nutmeg. Blend thoroughly.
4. Carefully fold the mixture into the cooled potatoes. Taste for salt. Garnish with a sprinkle with paprika.

Serves 8

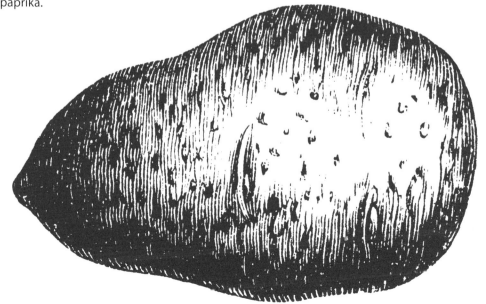

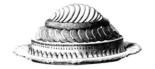

•HELEN WALKER•

Ratatouille Supreme

Rata - what? (rat-a-too-ee) This eggplant dish has an exotic name, but the flavor is nothing but down-home. It combines eggplant with zucchini and the usual suspects: onion, peppers and garlic. Tomatoes and fresh herbs lend their earthiness, while the wine adds a surprising depth of flavor. This dish is not one for the kindergartners, or maybe even middle-schoolers, but more mature palates will revel in the flavors. This dish takes a little effort, but you won't regret it! Try serving this with grilled Italian sausage and a little plain pasta on the side. Oooh – and garlic bread.

¹/₂ **cup olive oil**

4 cups eggplant, peeled and cubed into bite-sized pieces

4 cups zucchini, cubed

¹/₂ **cup bell pepper, cut into squares**

¹/₂ **cup onion, chopped**

2 tablespoons fresh garlic, chopped finely

¹/₂ **cup dry white wine**

4 fresh tomatoes, peeled and quartered (or one large can of whole tomatoes)

Pinch of thyme

1 bay leaf

1 teaspoon sweet basil

Pinch of rosemary

1 tablespoon salt

1 teaspoon white pepper

¹/₂ **cup pitted small black olives**

2 tablespoons chopped parsley

1. Preheat the oven to 350 degrees. Prepare a 3-quart casserole with non-stick spray.
2. Heat the oil in a large skillet or 8-quart pot. Sauté the eggplant and zucchini for 8 minutes, stirring frequently.
3. Add the peppers and onions. Cook, uncovered, for another 6 minutes.
4. Add the garlic and cook 2 minutes.
5. Stir in the wine, tomatoes, thyme, bay leaf, basil, rosemary, salt, pepper, and olives. Stir to blend completely. Taste and correct seasoning. Pour into the prepared casserole.
6. Bake, covered, for 20 minutes, or until the eggplant and zucchini are tender.
7. Sprinkle with the parsley and serve.

Serves 8

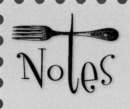

Notes

• *If you are using canned tomatoes, use whole ones, which have a better flavor than the pre-diced ones. Squeeze them in your hands to break them up before adding to the pot. I like to use fire-roasted tomatoes for the extra flavor.*

• *Try using the black pitted black olives from the deli section of the store rather than canned olives. The difference is very noticeable. Try some Kalamatas.*

• *As with most things Italian, this dish would be delicious with a splash of balsamic vinegar after it comes out of the oven. Make sure when you are using vinegar to finish a dish this way that it is of a high quality. A good aged balsamic will have an almost syrupy texture to it, with sweet overtones.*

• *This dish makes a fabulous topping for pasta. If you are using it as a sauce, loosen it up with an extra can of tomatoes and another splash of wine. Be sure to top with freshly-grated Parmesan and a grind of pepper.*

• *Use this for a stuffing in omelets or in a frittata. Don't forget the Parmesan. Finish with the chopped parsley.*

Easy Italian Spinach

This is the best and easiest spinach recipe ever. Try this even if you never have enjoyed spinach before. It is a long way from the taste and appearance of frozen, boxed spinach. A simple Italian preparation, it is vividly colored and takes just a minute or two to throw together. Silky smooth and fresh tasting, it is softened by the olive oil and perked up with the splash of vinegar. When you order spinach in Italy as a side dish, this is often the way it comes. It is perfect alongside any meat or creamy egg dish. Since the spinach cooks down so much, you will need to make several batches if you are preparing this for a lot of folks. It won't tempt the younger kids.

Per batch:
Olive oil
Butter
Garlic clove, peeled
Large bag of fresh baby spinach
Salt and pepper to taste
Balsamic vinegar

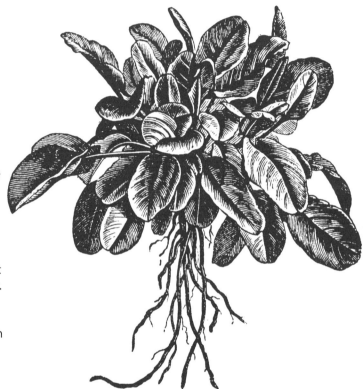

1. Film the bottom of a large sauté pan with olive oil. Use the largest pan you have because the raw spinach takes up a lot of room. Throw in a small pat of butter – you are just adding butter for the taste, and don't need much. Set the heat to medium high.
2. When the butter starts to melt, throw in the peeled garlic and cook for about a minute. You want to flavor the fat, not cook the garlic. Watch carefully; the garlic can burn quickly.
3. Dump the entire bag of spinach in the pan and let it sit for a little bit until the spinach on the bottom starts to wilt. Begin to move it around with tongs. Pull the wilted spinach up from the bottom and move the fresh spinach down closer to the heat.
4. Continue moving the spinach around until it has all wilted to about a quarter of its original volume. It will be a bright, jade green. Sprinkle with a little salt and continue moving it around. The whole process won't take much more than 5 minutes once the spinach starts to wilt.
5. Remove quickly to a serving plate and finish with a few grinds of black pepper and just a splash of balsamic vinegar. Be kind to your guests and remove the garlic clove before serving.

Serves 3-4

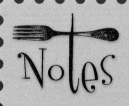

Notes

• *I like using both olive oil and butter when I sauté vegetables. The combination of flavors is better than either fat alone.*
• *You could prepare any green this way – turnip, kale, dandelion, chard, bok choy.*
• *This is a side that does not keep well for a long time. It is best served quickly.*

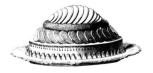

•DIANE ROBBINS•

Spinach Cheese Pie

The elegant pie, full of sharp cheese and spinach, is perfect for brunch! This is more of a grown-up recipe, what with all the green stuff so visible. There really is no way to make this interesting to children without eliminating the spinach. So save this one for a ladies' lunch or tailgate parties – it holds beautifully and tastes wonderful at room temperature. Do try making it in a frozen pie crust as a delicious variation.

1 package chopped spinach, defrosted and drained

12 ounces cottage cheese

³/₄ stick (6 tablespoons) unsalted butter, cut in chunks

12 ounces sharp cheddar Cracker Barrel cheese, grated

6 eggs, beaten lightly

1. Toss all the ingredients together and pour into two 9-inch pie pans.
2. Bake for 45-60 minutes at 350 degrees.
3. Serve immediately.

Serves 6-8

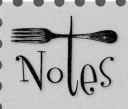

Notes

• *This makes a very rich dish. To save on calories and fat, cut down the butter to just 2 tablespoons. You will still have that butter taste and the texture won't be significantly affected.*

• *Try baking this in a pie crust – it is delicious! Just pour the mixture into a frozen crust and bake.*

• *To garnish, set aside about ¹/₄ - ¹/₂ cup of the cheese and sprinkle on top.*

• *You can use fresh spinach instead of frozen, if you prefer. Sauté two large bunches of spinach in a large skillet filmed with olive oil. Cook on medium high until the spinach wilts and reduces. Remove cooked spinach to a colander and press out as much liquid as possible before adding to the rest of the ingredients.*

• *I always like to add a pinch of cayenne to this sort of dish. You could also add just a pinch of nutmeg for another layer of flavor. And garlic goes with everything! If you are using fresh spinach, add a little minced garlic to the sauté pan; if you use frozen spinach, sprinkle in ¹/₂ teaspoon of garlic powder into the egg mixture.*

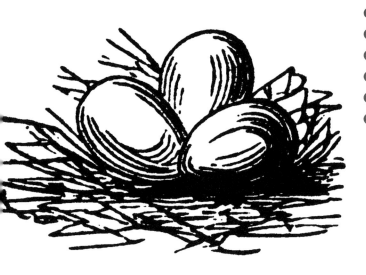

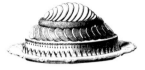

·MIKE FIELDS, FLAT CREEK RANCH·

Confetti Rice

This deceptively simple dish is more like a creamy risotto, minus the careful stirring. Instead of cooking the rice completely on top of the stove, it is baked with the vegetables. The result is delectable. We first encountered it at Flat Creek Ranch in Jackson, Wyoming. Mike Fields, an inspired cook, prepared memorable meals every night, and this was one of our favorite dishes. He shared this simple recipe readily, noting how easy it is to vary the vegetables. He likes using root vegetables, like onions and carrots, combined with deeply flavored mushrooms. Use what you have on hand, or what compliments the entrée you are serving.

3 tablespoons butter

1¹/₂ cup chopped onions

1 cup carrots, cut into 1-inch dice

8 ounces mushrooms (portabella preferred) cleaned and chopped in a large dice

1 cup celery, finely chopped

1 clove of garlic, minced

2 cups rice

2 cups broth (see Notes)

2 cups water

1 teaspoon salt, divided

¹/₂ teaspoon white pepper

1. Preheat the oven to 350 degrees. Treat a large casserole with non-stick spray.
2. Melt the butter in a large skillet. When if foams, add the onions, carrots, celery and garlic. Cook for five minutes until the vegetables begin to soften.
3. Add the mushrooms, ¹/₂ teaspoon salt and the pepper to the pan and continue cooking the vegetables until the mushrooms release their liquid. Cook a bit longer until some of the moisture evaporates.
4. Meanwhile, bring the stock and water and ¹/₂ teaspoon salt to boil in a large pot. When boiling, add the rice and boil, uncovered, for 2-3 minutes.
5. Add the vegetables, reduce heat and stir well to combine.
6. Pour the mixture into the prepared casserole and bake, covered, for 20 minutes. Uncover and check that the rice is tender and the moisture has been absorbed. If not, bake, covered, another 10 minutes.
7. Remove and serve hot.

Serve 6-8

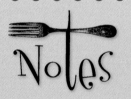

Notes

- *These proportions make a dish long on rice and short on vegetables; it eats like a starch, not a vegetable. Feel free to increase the amount of vegetables you use, either by adding more of the same (I like extra mushrooms) or choosing an addition. Eggplant, summer squash and zucchini, asparagus and broccoli would all make delicious additions.*
- *This makes a very mild dish that receives gravies and sauces beautifully. It could just as easily be a sparky little side dish with the addition of stronger spices. The idea is to season the vegetables well before adding them to the rice, so you have the two notes of mild and intense rather than everything tasting the same in each bite. You could use a teaspoon of Cajun seasoning or Italian seasoning (especially wonderful if eggplant is one of your add-ins), or just throw in a little cayenne pepper. There are always jalapenos in my fridge waiting for a chance to shine, and they would be good, as would a can of milder chiles. Check out some of the spice mixes at Penzey's (see ingredients chapter).This is one of those dishes that can go many, many ways.*
- *You can use homemade stock or prepared canned broth in whatever flavor will compliment your meal: chicken, beef, or vegetable. If you are using regular canned broth, taste the broth/water mix before adding the rice. Some canned broths are very salty.*
- *You can substitute black pepper if you don't have white, but white is the best – fragrant, slightly floral, and it disappears in the white rice.*
- *Try and keep all your vegetables cut into similar sizes so they look nice and cook evenly.*
- *Mike cautioned not to substitute oil for the butter. As the dish cools, the butter won't pool the way oil does.*
- *A sprinkle of freshly chopped parsley would make a delightful garnish sprinkled on after the rice is removed from the oven.*

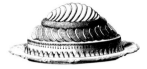

·KATHY HALL·

Butternut Squash Casserole

This colorful casserole works well as a side dish if you are serving a Thanksgiving menu – a favorite of high schoolers. It is flavorful, thanks to the spices, and sweet – but not too sweet (it doesn't taste like a pie filling.) The younger kids will go for it since it has all those marshmallows and the sugar. Of course, it works beautifully with roasted meats of any sort. Best of all, it is easy to prepare, especially if you use frozen, pureed squash. A winner!

2 cups butternut squash, cooked and mashed
3 tablespoons butter, melted
$^3/_4$ cup sugar
$^1/_3$ cup milk
$^1/_2$ teaspoon salt
$^1/_4$ teaspoon cinnamon
$^1/_4$ teaspoon nutmeg
3 eggs, beaten until fluffy
1 teaspoon vanilla
Miniature marshmallows

1. Preheat oven to 325 degrees. Prepare a round casserole dish with non-stick spray.
2. Combine butter, sugar, milk, salt, cinnamon and nutmeg with the mashed squash. Mix well.
3. Beat the eggs until light and fluffy. Add the vanilla. Fold carefully into the squash mixture.
4. Pour mixture into the prepared casserole and sprinkle with the marshmallows, covering the surface completely.
5. Bake approximately 1 hour, or until the marshmallows are lightly browned and the casserole is bubbly.

Serves 6-8

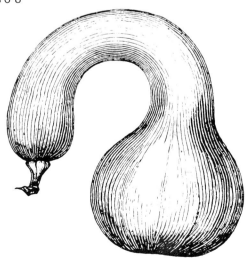

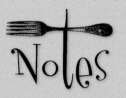

Notes

• Butternut squash can be intimidating, but it doesn't need to be. Don't try to peel it while it is raw – you will give up on this recipe if you do! Simply cut the squash in half and scrape out the seeds. Pierce each half several times with a toothpick. Oil a large baking dish and place the squash on it, flesh side up. Lightly oil the surface of the squash. Roast for 45-60 minutes in a 375 degree oven until the flesh gives easily when pressed with a spoon. Cool and then scoop the cooked squash out of the shell. It will mash easily now.
• Or – avoid the whole scraping, piercing, scooping exercise and buy frozen butternut squash, already mashed! I have seen it in the freezer at our Whole Foods grocery store.
• If you have an aversion to marshmallows, simply eliminate them. Try a mixture of chopped pecans and brown sugar, instead. Use about 1 – 1$^1/_2$ cups chopped pecans (depending on the casserole you use – make enough to cover the surface of the dish generously) and 2-3 tablespoons of brown sugar. Mmmm.
•You could make this dish with sweet potatoes instead. Simply substitute cooked mashed sweet potatoes for the squash; everything else remains the same.

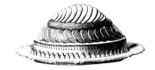

•SHIRLEY JARVIS•

Traditional cornbread stuffing

The secret to this recipe is to spread the dressing out in a shallow pan so that it gets crispy on top as it bakes. Softened with a little gravy and a bite of cranberry sauce, it is heaven! This is an easy recipe that goes together quickly, and it tastes like it came from grandma's house.

1 cup chopped celery

1 cup chopped onion

1 tablespoon rubbed sage (or more to taste)

3 cups turkey or chicken broth (canned or homemade)

$^1/_2$ - $^2/_3$ stick butter

1 small package Pepperidge Farm Herb dressing mix

8 cornbread muffins (easy recipe next page), broken into large pieces

1. Preheat the oven to 425 degrees. Prepare a baking sheet with non-stick spray or butter.
2. In a small sauce pan, mix broth, butter, celery, onion, and sage. Simmer until vegetables are soft.
3. Pour the mixture over the crumbled corn muffins and dressing mix. Combine thoroughly. If more moisture is needed, add a little canola oil and hot water.
4. Spread thin in a large greased baking sheet and bake for about 20-25 minutes until it begins to turn brown and the edges are crispy.

Serves 6-8

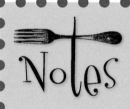

Notes

• The recipe calls for rubbed sage, but you could substitute poultry spice if that is all you have.
• You shouldn't need any added salt since the dressing and cornbread mix are already seasoned. But taste before baking to be sure.

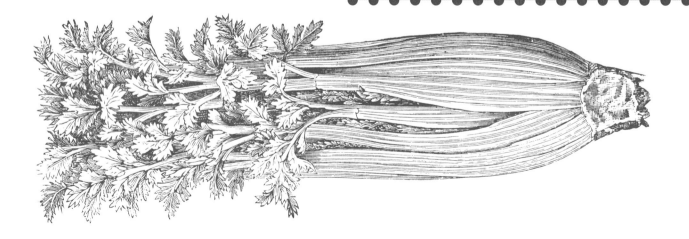

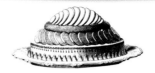

•SHIRLEY JARVIS•

cornbread muffins

1¹/₂ **cups Three Rivers cornmeal mix**

1 teaspoon sugar

1 egg

Enough buttermilk to make a stiff, moist batter

1. Preheat the oven to 425 degrees. Put a few drops of canola oil in the bottom of an 8-cup muffin pan. Put the pan in the oven while it preheats.
2. Combine all the batter ingredients and spoon into the hot muffin cups.
3. Bake 20-25 minutes, until nicely browned.

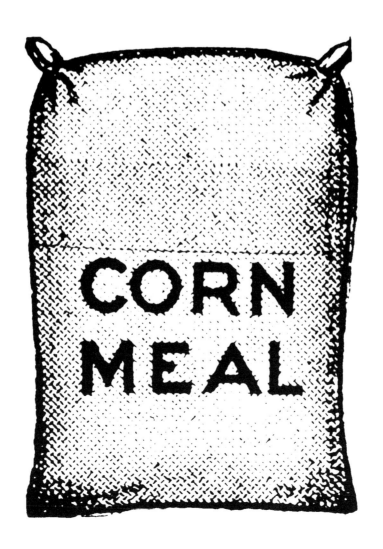

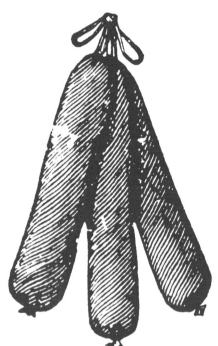

stuffing with a Kick

This is the stuffing I make every Thanksgiving, served with Mexican cranberries. It is chock full of cornbread, chiles, roasted garlic, sausage and pecans. There are several steps to making this, so plan enough time. This is an assertive stuffing, yet not so hot it hurts. You can control the level of heat easily. Young kids probably won't go for this, but its complex flavors go well with roast chicken or pork as well as turkey. It is delicious hot, room temperature, or cold from the refrigerator right out of the dish. It makes wonderful sandwiches with sliced smoked turkey from the deli and a little cranberry sauce.

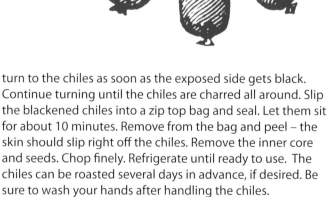

Cornbread – 2 batches, made without sugar

Entire head of garlic

Olive oil

2 fresh poblano chiles

1 pound hot breakfast sausage

1 can chopped green chiles, well drained

1-2 cups pecans, toasted and chopped

1 large head of cilantro, or more to taste,   loosely chopped

Butter (unsalted) – about 1 stick

2 cups chopped onion (2 medium onions), medium dice

2 cups (4-5 stalks) chopped celery, medium dice

1 tablespoon plus 1 teaspoon poultry seasoning or to taste

1 teaspoon chipotle chili powder (optional but highly recommended)

Salt, pepper to taste

1 – 2 cans chicken broth (about 3 cups if using homemade)

2 eggs

1. Make two batches of cornbread, using your favorite recipe or mix. You might not use all of both batches. It will depend on how moist or spicy you want your dressing. The more cornbread you use, the less spicy your final product will be.
2. Cut the tip off an entire head of garlic, exposing the upper portion of all the cloves. Place the garlic head on a piece of tinfoil and drizzle with about a teaspoon of olive oil. Sprinkle lightly with salt. Seal the tinfoil and bake in a 375 oven for about 30 minutes, until the garlic is roasted and soft. After it cools a bit, squeeze the soft roasted garlic out of each clove into a small bowl. Mash the roasted garlic until it is smooth (you will discover any bits of the skin that snuck in). Add about $1/4$ cup chicken broth to make a thinner, pourable mixture. Set aside.
3. Turn the oven to broil and blacken the poblano chiles. Lay them on a sheet of tin foil and place the foil on a cookie sheet. Place the oven rack on the top setting, close to the heat element. Roast the chiles, watching closely. Give a $1/4$

turn to the chiles as soon as the exposed side gets black. Continue turning until the chiles are charred all around. Slip the blackened chiles into a zip top bag and seal. Let them sit for about 10 minutes. Remove from the bag and peel – the skin should slip right off the chiles. Remove the inner core and seeds. Chop finely. Refrigerate until ready to use. The chiles can be roasted several days in advance, if desired. Be sure to wash your hands after handling the chiles.

4. Brown the sausage, breaking it up into crumbles while it cooks. Cook until dry and crispy; drain well.
5. Toast the pecans in a skillet over medium high heat, being careful no to let them burn.
6. Chop cilantro coarsely.
7. Melt 3 tablespoons of butter in a large skillet. Sauté 1 cup each onion and celery (leaving one cup each raw). Cook until softened and translucent, about 10 minutes.

continued on page 137

continued from page 136

TO ASSEMBLE:

1. Treat a large casserole with non-stick spray. Preheat the oven to 350 degrees.
2. Break cornbread into chunks in a very large bowl. Use about $^3/_4$ of the entire amount, keeping a little on the side to add if you get the mixture too wet at some point. If you end up using it all, you might need to increase your spices.
3. Add the canned chiles, blackened chiles, roasted garlic mixture, sausage, pecans, cooked onions and celery, raw onions and celery, and chopped cilantro.
4. Mix well and moisten with 1 can of chicken broth, tossing carefully.
5. Beat two eggs until foamy and light. Melt the rest of the butter. Pour each over the cornbread mixture.
6. Season with the poultry seasoning (adding more or less to taste – taste as you go – this is critical!), chipotle powder if using (I like at least 1 teaspoon), salt and pepper. Since your cornbread was seasoned when you baked it, you shouldn't need much. Start with 1 teaspoon and taste.
7. If your mixture isn't moist enough (this will depend on the amount of cornbread you use), add more chicken broth until you reach the desired consistency. It should be sticky (holding its shape when you mound it), since it dries out as it cooks.
8. Spoon the mixture into the large casserole. Cover and cook for about 30 minutes. Uncover and continue cooking for another 30 minutes.

12 generous servings

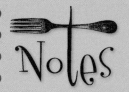

Notes

- *Try making the cornbread with buttermilk for even more flavor in the stuffing. And, if it doesn't bother you, use bacon fat instead of oil in the cornbread recipe – it adds a terrific smoky accent.*
- *I like to use my hands to combine all the ingredients for this dish. It seems to be easier to blend things without breaking up the cornbread too much. I can feel if there are any dry pockets when adding the liquids. Just be sure to wash your hands well when you are done since you will be handling chiles.*
- *Taste, taste, taste as you go. If your cornbread is well-salted, you won't need to add a lot of extra salt to the final dish. If your chiles happen to be especially potent, you might not need as much chili powder.*
- *Add or subtract at will: leave out the nuts or sausage. Use parsley instead of cilantro, if you are not a fan. Use either the green chiles or the roasted poblanos instead of both if you are nervous. The green chiles are very mild and add flavor rather than heat. The poblanos have a little more kick – but not much. Just be sure you remove all the seeds, which is where the heat lives, and you won't feel a burn. Certainly avoid the chipotle chili powder to cut down on heat.*
- *If you want to skip roasting the garlic (which adds a deep, earthy flavor), you could sauté 4-5 finely chopped cloves in the butter when you sauté the onions and celery. Or, you could use about 1 teaspoon powdered garlic when adding your other dry seasonings.*
- *Do take the time to toast the pecans – it makes a big difference in their flavor.*
- *This can be made ahead lots of different ways. Make the cornbread 2-3 days before assembling, as well as the roasted chiles and roasted garlic. The sausage can be browned ahead of time as well. Or prepare all parts of the recipe and assemble on the same day and let it marinate in the fridge for 2-3 days before cooking and serving it. Or bake it and then freeze it.*

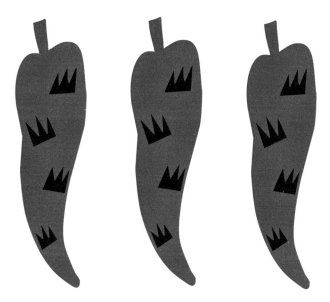

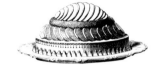

•MAUREEN ROWAN•

Tomato Tart

This is as simple – and delicious! – as it gets. It is the perfect combination of flavors – tomatoes and fresh basil held together with cheese. That's it! No elaborate sauces or preparation. Maureen is an accomplished cook and this is one of her lucky family's favorite dishes. Try it as a vegetarian entrée, or a wonderful accompaniment beside a light chicken dish. It works for a tailgate at room temperature. It could also star in a breakfast buffet with bacon or sausage on the side, biscuits and fresh fruit.

1 basic pie shell, either frozen, or refrigerator dough

8 ounces shredded mozzarella cheese

2 heaping tablespoons fresh, chopped basil

4-5 ripe Roma tomatoes sliced $^1/_2$ inch thick

$^1/_2$ teaspoon salt

$^1/_4$ teaspoon pepper

$^1/_4$ cup extra virgin olive oil

1. Preheat oven to 400 degrees.
2. If you are using refrigerated pie dough, spread the dough into a pie plate and press into place.
3. Cover the bottom of the shell evenly with the shredded cheese. Sprinkle with basil. Layer the sliced tomatoes over the basil, filling in all the space as evenly as possible. Season the tomatoes with olive oil, salt and freshly ground black pepper.
4. Bake 30-40 minutes, until the crust is golden and the cheese is bubbly. Slice into wedges. This can be served hot or at room temperature.

Serves 4-6

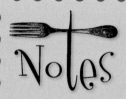

Notes

• *Try and use the small, pear-shaped Roma tomatoes for this recipe. They have less juice and hold their shape beautifully when cooked. If you do use a different tomato, slice and drain on paper towels for a few minutes before adding to the tart.*

• *If you wanted to gussy up this dish, you could finish with a sprinkle of nutty, freshly grated Parmesan cheese.*

• *You can also embellish the filling (although it doesn't need it!) with some Italian standbys like sliced black olives, sautéed mushrooms, or sliced artichoke hearts. You could also sprinkle some crispy pancetta or bacon over the cheese before adding the tomatoes.*

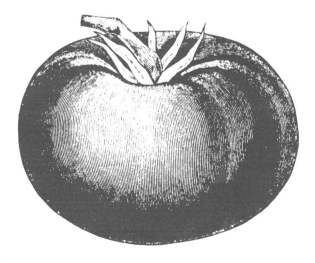

RECiPES

SALADS

Fruit Salads

Vegetable Salads

Entrée Salads

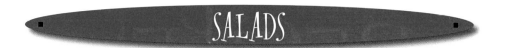
Fruit Salads

Mexican Cranberries

This is my family's favorite cranberry sauce. The sweet and hot combination is irresistible! I have served it for years at Thanksgiving with Dressing with a Kick, but it makes a wonderful condiment for sandwiches, say – smoked turkey and brie on focaccia. Or spoon it on top of cream cheese and serve with crackers.

1 16-ounce can whole berry cranberry sauce

1 10$^{1}/_{2}$ ounce jar jalapeno pepper jelly

2 tablespoons chopped fresh cilantro

1. Combine the cranberry sauce and jelly in a small saucepan; cook over low heat, stirring often, until jelly melts. Cool.
2. Gently stir in the chopped fresh cilantro. Chill until ready to serve.

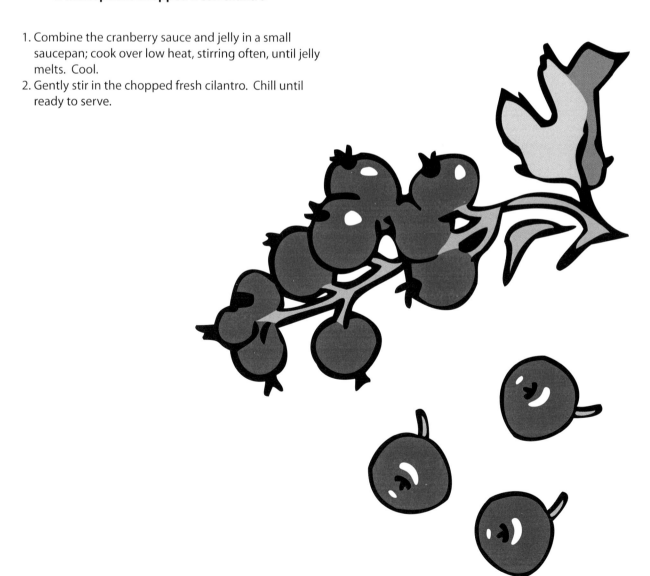

Fruit Salads

•SHIRLEY JARVIS•

Mom's Cranberry Salad

This classic cranberry salad will keep in the refrigerator from Thanksgiving to Christmas. It may also be frozen. It combines the flavors of cranberries and oranges in a molded salad. Try serving it over a bit of cottage cheese with a dollop of mayonnaise and saltines for a light lunch or dinner. The orange peel in this salad gives it a bright bite that is refreshing.

2 small boxes of cherry Jell-O

2^1/$_2$ cups boiling water

2 pounds fresh cranberries

2 oranges with peel

1 cup white sugar

1. Dissolve Jell-O in boiling water; set aside to cool. Do NOT let it set.
2. Wash and cull the cranberries. Quarter the oranges and remove seeds and white core; cut into smaller pieces.
3. Use a blender or food processor to cut cranberries and oranges into very small pieces; do not leave any large pieces of orange peel.
4. Mix the fruit with the sugar, stirring until the sugar is dissolved. Stir into the cooled Jell-O. Refrigerate until set.

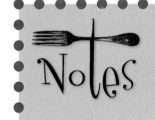

Notes

For a delicious variation, try adding pecans, finely chopped apple, pineapple, and/or celery, according to taste. Start with half a cup of the ingredient and add more if desired.

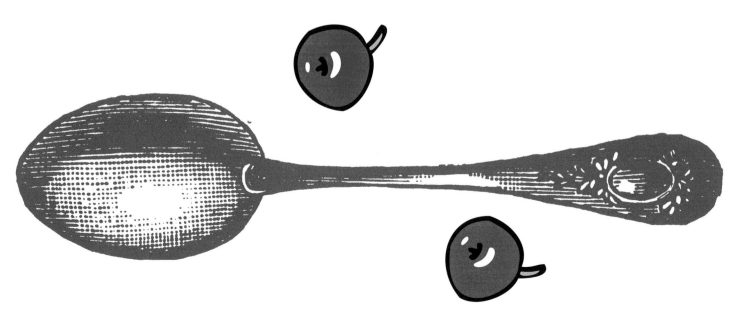

Fruit Salads

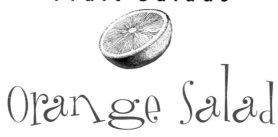

Orange Salad

This one has been in my family for years. I have no idea how old it is, but it is a favorite. Pineapple and oranges are nestled in a mixture of nuts, sour cream and Jell-O. Rich, colorful, easy to fix, it can be made ahead. Kids like the Jell-O aspect. A classic!

1 large box of orange Jell-O

$^1/_3$ cup sugar

1 cup hot water

1 large can crushed pineapple, undrained

1 cup mandarin oranges, undrained

2 cups sour cream

$^3/_4$ cup toasted pecans

1. Combine Jell-O mix and sugar in a large bowl. Add the hot water and stir until dissolved.
2. Add the pineapple and oranges, mixing well. Cool in the refrigerator for about 15 minutes.
3. Fold in the sour cream and nuts, stirring to distribute all the solids evenly through the gelatin. Refrigerate for at least 4 hours.

Serves 6-8

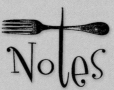

Notes

• This dish is pretty in a decorative mold. You can use a circle mold and fill the center with extra sour cream, green grapes for contrast, or flowers.
• If you don't have a large platter, cover a stout piece of cardboard with tin foil.
• To loosen the dish from the mold, set the bottom of the mold in hot water for about 15 seconds and then flip onto the serving platter.
• Toasted pecans make a big difference and are easy to do: heat a heavy skillet over medium heat and add the pecans. Shake the pan occasionally until the nuts begin to brown. Watch closely, because once the nuts start to cook, they will burn quickly.
• This recipe is easy to double.

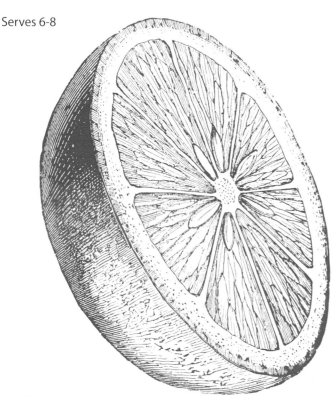

Fruit Salads

·DIANE ROBBINS·

Pink Lady Frozen Salad

Oooh, Ladies' Lunch! Teacher Appreciation lunch. These frozen fruit muffins, full of nuts, cherries and whipped cream, can be made ahead, ready to go when needed. They compliment almost any menu. This is a great way to get children to ingest fruit. You could even use this as a dessert with a nice lemony cookie on the side.

- **1 21-ounce can cherry pie filling**
- **1 20-ounce can crushed pineapple, drained**
- **3-4 bananas, mashed**
- **1 cup chopped nuts, toasted**
- **1 14-ounce can sweetened condensed milk**
- **12 ounces frozen whipped topping**

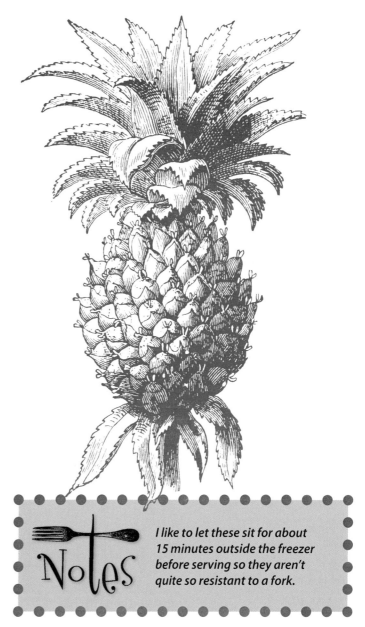

1. Combine the fruits, nuts and condensed milk in a large bowl.
2. Carefully fold in the whipped topping.
3. Spoon into muffin tins lined with paper cups and freeze. Or pour into a rectangular baking pan treated with non-stick spray.
4. Once frozen, store the muffins in a zip top bag in the freezer until ready to serve.

Makes 2 dozen muffins

Notes

I like to let these sit for about 15 minutes outside the freezer before serving so they aren't quite so resistant to a fork.

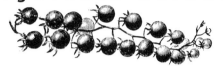

SALADS

Vegetable Salads

•LEN POUSSON•

Avocado Salsa

This recipe will work well for teenagers and adults – and some younger kids. Nothing too spicy – but it IS green. It is more like a chopped salad, since the avocados are not mashed as with a guacamole. This makes a terrific side for a Mexican themed menu that might include enchiladas, build-your-own tacos, tamale pie or a Mexican chicken casserole. Or use it as a side for grilled meat, especially pork chops. It requires overnight marinating and can be made several days ahead before adding the avocados.

1 can (17-ounce) corn, drained

2 cans (2^{1}/4 ounces each) sliced ripe olives, drained

1 red bell pepper, diced

^{1}/2 small red onion, diced very fine

1 clove garlic, minced

^{1}/3 cup olive oil

^{1}/4 cup lemon juice

3 tablespoons white wine vinegar

1 teaspoon oregano

^{1}/2 teaspoon salt

^{1}/2 teaspoon pepper

4 medium avocados

^{1}/2 cup cilantro, chopped (optional)

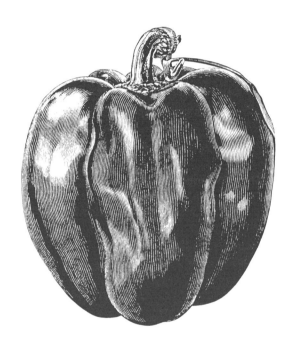

1. In a large bowl, combine corn, olives, and bell pepper.
2. In a separate bowl, combine onion, minced garlic, oil, lemon juice, vinegar, oregano, salt, and pepper. Mix well. Pour over corn mixture and toss to coat.
3. Cover and refrigerate overnight.
4. Just before serving, peel avocados and remove the pit. Chop and add to salsa along with the cilantro, if using. Toss gently, coating the avocados thoroughly. Serve chilled.

Serves 6-8

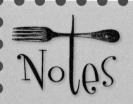

Notes

• *Try using a meaty olive like a Kalamata from the gourmet section of the deli, for a delightful flavor boost for grown-ups. Be sure to use the optional cilantro. A dash of chipotle chili powder couldn't hurt, either!*
• *This would be a great companion for cheese quesadillas on an appetizer platter.*

SALADS

Vegetable Salads

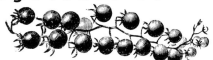

•LEN POUSSON•

Black Bean & Avocado Salad

This is spicy delicious. The combination of black beans and avocados is pretty adult-tasting, so skip this one if serving younger children. It makes a wonderful side dish for a Mexican-themed menu, but can just as easily be served with grilled meat, especially pork. It makes a great vegetarian main dish salad, too.

Grated zest of 1 lime

1 tablespoon fresh lime juice

$^1/_2$ teaspoon sugar

$^1/_2$ teaspoon pure ground dried chiles, such as ancho, or regular chili powder

1 garlic clove, crushed through a press

$^1/_3$ cup extra-virgin olive oil

One 15- to 19-ounce can black beans, drained and rinsed

$^1/_3$ cup finely chopped red onion

1 ripe Hass avocado, pitted, peeled, and cut into $^1/_2$-inch dice

1 vinegar-packed roasted red bell pepper, seeds and ribs removed, cut into 1-inch dice

Salt and freshly ground black pepper to taste

1. To make the dressing, pulse the lime zest and juice, sugar, ground chiles, and garlic in a blender to combine. With the blender on, gradually add the oil through the top vent. Transfer to a medium bowl.
2. Add the beans, red onion, avocado, and bell pepper to the dressing and toss gently to evenly distribute the dressing. Season with salt and pepper.
3. Cover and refrigerate until chilled, about 2 hours, before serving.

Serves 4

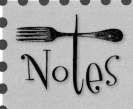

Notes

• *The salad can be made up to two days ahead. Combine everything but the avocado, which is added just before serving. Season with additional lime juice, salt, and pepper.*

• *If you are making this a vegetarian dish, try adding about 8 ounces of cubed sharp cheddar cheese. More protein and lots of extra flavor.*

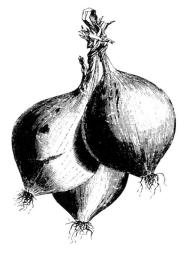

Vegetable Salads

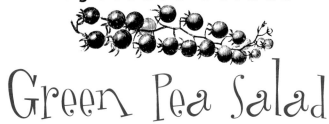

Green Pea Salad

This is a delightful little salad that works well on a buffet. The crunch of the cucumber, the tang of sour cream and the lift of fresh dill distinguish this colorful pea salad. Fast and easy to make, it will please the adults more than little kids.

1 pound frozen petite green peas

1 cup diced cucumber

1 clove garlic, minced

$^1/_4$ cup fresh dill, chopped

1 red bell pepper, chopped

1 onion, chopped & sautéed until translucent

$^2/_3$ cup sour cream

$^1/_3$ cup mayonnaise

2 tablespoons fresh lemon juice

Salt and white pepper to taste

1. Thaw peas and drain well.
2. Combine all ingredients in a large bowl. Stir well to coat all vegetables.
3. Chill until ready to serve.

Serves 4-6

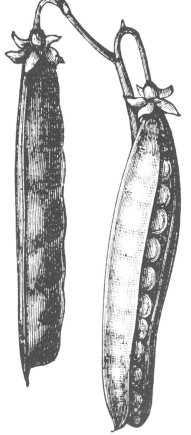

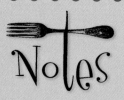

Notes

• *Sauté the onions in a little olive oil and let them cool before adding to the other ingredients.*
• *Cut the cucumber and bell pepper into uniform size pieces for a pretty salad.*
• *Don't substitute dried dill for fresh.*
• *You could use black pepper in this dish, but the milder white pepper is a little more inconspicuous and flowery, which complements the fresh herb flavor. Small details like this make a difference.*

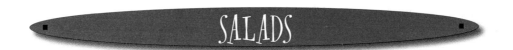

Vegetable Salads

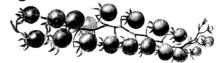

•SHIRLEY JARVIS•

Sour Cream Cucumber Salad

This is absolutely the quickest, easiest – and most delicious! - make-ahead summer salad ever. It also travels well for tailgating or covered dish affairs. When you make it ahead, the vinegar permeates the cucumbers in a very yummy way. The sour cream smoothes out the vinegar's tartness and the sugar balances it. It is just a treat of textures and tastes.

1 teaspoon salt

1 tablespoon vinegar

3 heaping tablespoons sour cream

1 tablespoon sugar

4-5 small cucumbers, peeled and sliced

1 medium red onion, peeled and sliced

Dash of pepper for garnish

1. Mix together salt, vinegar, sour cream, sugar.
2. Fold in the onions and cucumbers and refrigerate until well-chilled.

Serves 4-6

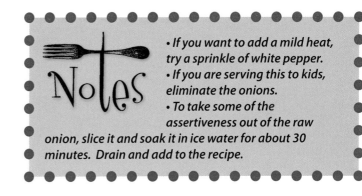

Notes

• *If you want to add a mild heat, try a sprinkle of white pepper.*
• *If you are serving this to kids, eliminate the onions.*
• *To take some of the assertiveness out of the raw onion, slice it and soak it in ice water for about 30 minutes. Drain and add to the recipe.*

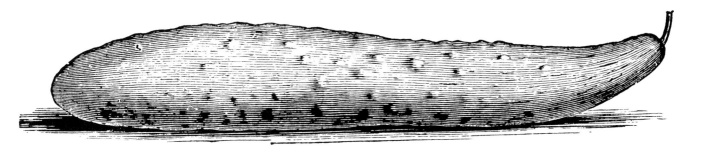

Vegetable Salads

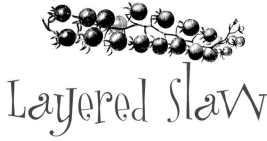

Layered Slaw

This salad is refreshing and quite a hit with the older crowd. Younger kids won't be thrilled with the whole notion of cabbage, so there isn't much point in trying to kid-friendly this one up. It is a good make-ahead dish since it needs to sit at least 8 hours. It gets better after 24 hours. It is especially good with roasted meats and barbecue, since it is similar to a slaw. Instead of mayonnaise, it has the tang of olives, Feta and a vinaigrette.

1 medium onion, peeled and thinly sliced

1 small cabbage, shredded

2 tomatoes, cut into wedges

1 small yellow bell pepper, cut into thin strips

$^1/_2$ cup sliced ripe olives

$^3/_4$ cup crumbled Feta cheese

$^2/_3$ cup olive oil

$^1/_3$ cup red wine vinegar

2 cloves garlic, minced

1 teaspoon ground cumin

$^3/_4$ teaspoon salt

$^1/_2$ teaspoon pepper

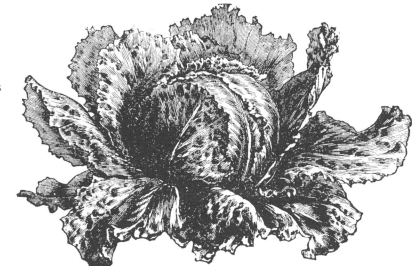

1. Halve each onion slice and separate.
2. Combine the onion, cabbage, tomatoes, pepper, olives and cheese in a large bowl that can be covered tightly; set aside.
3. Combine the olive oil, vinegar, garlic, cumin, salt, and pepper in a jar. Shake well until the ingredients are well blended.
4. Pour dressing over the salad; mix well.
5. Cover and refrigerate for at least 8 hours. Toss before serving.

6-8 servings

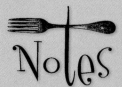

Notes

• *Use Feta that is packed in liquid rather than the pre-crumbled cheese. The flavor will be better. Feel free to experiment with flavored Fetas, too.*
• *If you want to avoid garlic nightmares, make the dressing a day ahead. Cut the cloves of garlic in half and leave them in the vinaigrette and let the ingredients steep with the garlic. When ready to assemble, toss the garlic and pour the dressing.*

Vegetable Salads

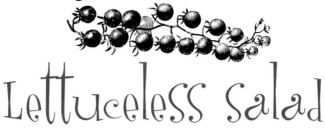

Lettuceless Salad

This recipe has a long ingredient list, but it is one terrific salad. The combination of vegetables, cheese and fruit with a tangy herb dressing is so unusual. And popular – with the adults (this is not a young-kid favorite). Someone always asks for this recipe when I take it to an event. You'll get more dressing than you need with this recipe, so use the extra on steamed veggies or on top of a baked potato. This is a good vegetarian offering.

HERB DRESSING (makes 3¹/₂ cups)

1 egg

1 tablespoon white vinegar
(or other mild vinegar like rice or cider)

2 teaspoons Dijon mustard

1 small garlic clove, halved

1 teaspoon dill seed

1 teaspoon salt

¹/₂ teaspoon dried thyme,

¹/₂ teaspoon marjoram

¹/₂ teaspoon basil

¹/₂ teaspoon celery salt

¹/₂ teaspoon ground white pepper (no substitute)

¹/₂ cup canola or olive oil

1 cup buttermilk

2 cups mayonnaise, Hellmann's preferred

SALAD

1 head broccoli, cut into florets

1 head cauliflower, cut into florets

1 pound cheddar cheese, cut into small cubes

4 celery stalks, sliced

3 large carrots, sliced

1 cucumber, cut into large cubes

1 red apple, unpeeled, cored and cut into cubes

1 small onion, large dice

1 green bell pepper, seeded and sliced or diced

¹/₃ cup raisins

1 cup salted roasted sunflower seeds

12 generous side-dish servings

For the dressing:
1. Combine egg, vinegar, mustard, garlic, dill seed, salt, thyme, marjoram, basil, celery salt and pepper in a processor and blend well.
2. With the machine running, pour oil and then buttermilk through the feed tube slowly until the mixture thickens.
3. Transfer to a large bowl and whisk in mayonnaise. Set aside.

For the salad:
1. Combine all the ingredients except the sunflower seeds in a large bowl. Pour one cup of the dressing over the vegetables and mix well.
2. If serving individually, spoon servings onto salad plate and garnish with seeds. Pass additional dressing.
3. If serving on a buffet, add more dressing until you have it as wet as you like. You won't need the entire recipe. Serve extra dressing on the side. Top with the sunflower seeds at the last minute.

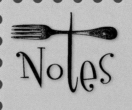

Notes

• Cut all the salad ingredients about the same size so no one flavor dominates another. Plus, it makes a prettier presentation.
• The raw egg can be eliminated, if desired.
• Fresh herbs would be a wonderful substitute for the dried. You need three times as much of a fresh herb as a dried one for the same amount of flavoring, so use 1¹/₂ teaspoons of chopped fresh herbs. You could add some fresh dill, too, if you have it – about 1 teaspoon, chopped. Don't fret if you are missing one of the called for herbs. You could substitute or just leave it out – there are so many other flavors going on it won't have a huge effect.

Vegetable Salads

Arugula Salad With Cranberries & Walnuts

This salad was inspired by one of our favorites at a local restaurant. The combination of chewy dried cranberries, toasted walnuts, salty olives and creamy Feta cheese is set off to perfection with a simple drizzle of fine-quality olive oil. This salad is easy to assemble on-site at a potluck or fix quickly at home for instant dinner. It is a wonderful vegetarian offering, with high quality protein in the nuts and cheese. Or, add some strips of grilled chicken for a complete meal.

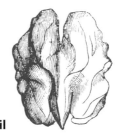
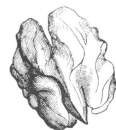

Baby arugula lettuce

Dried cranberries

Toasted walnuts

Feta cheese, crumbled

Kalamata olives

Fresh herbs (optional) such as parsley, oregano, cilantro, chives, basil

High quality olive oil

Salt and freshly ground black pepper

1. Toast walnuts in a pan over medium high heat. Watch them carefully; they burn easily. Set aside to cool.
2. To assemble the salad: in a large bowl, or on individual chilled salad plates, layer the desired amount of arugula. Add chopped fresh herbs if you are using them. Sprinkle with salt and a grind of pepper.
3. Scatter the cranberries and walnuts in desired amount. I like a generous tablespoon of each. Mound crumbled Feta cheese in the center and finish with 3-4 olives per plate. Drizzle lightly with olive oil and a final grind of pepper.
4. Serve immediately.

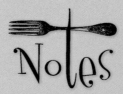

Notes

• *Be sure to use baby arugula lettuce leaves. More mature leaves are bitter.*
• *You can use any mix of baby greens if you don't like the tartness of arugula. The pre-washed and bagged mix of greens is a great time-saver.*
• *You can use any fruit and nut combination that strikes your fancy: strawberries and pecans; blueberries or raspberries and almonds; dried cherries and cashews; pine nuts and any berry.*
• *It is imperative to use a fine-quality olive oil in this recipe since it is the only dressing ingredient. Choose a light, fruity green oil or a rich, golden Greek oil.*
• *If you want to up the healthy quotient of this already healthful salad, don't toast the nuts. Heat destroys some of the healthy oils found in nuts (but intensifies the flavor.)*
• *If serving at a buffet, before adding the other ingredients, drizzle the salad with oil and toss well to coat all the leaves. Finally, add and evenly distribute the other ingredients. Always finish with a grind of black pepper!*

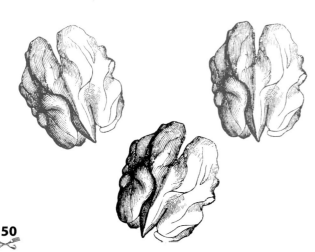

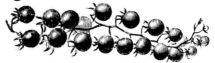

Vegetable Salads

•WEBB FRIDAY NIGHT FEASTS•

Mandarin Salad

This recipe has been a Friday night favorite for the football team's pre-game dinner for years. It is equally good for an elegant dinner for adults. This colorful lettuce salad has the crunch of celery and almonds with the interesting contrast of sweet oranges and tangy sweet/sour dressing. It goes well with any entrée, especially pork. These directions are geared toward a mobile preparation – perfect for a tailgate or potluck.

SALAD

^{1}/$_4$ **cup sliced almonds**

1^1/$_2$ **tablespoons sugar**

^{1}/$_2$ **head iceberg lettuce, torn into pieces**

^{1}/$_2$ **head Romaine lettuce, torn into pieces**

1 cup chopped celery

2 green onions, thinly sliced

1 11-ounce can of mandarin oranges, drained and chilled

DRESSING

^{1}/$_2$ **teaspoon salt**

^{1}/$_2$ **teaspoon pepper**

2 tablespoons sugar

2 tablespoons vinegar

^{1}/$_4$ **cup good quality olive oil**

Dash of Tabasco sauce

1 tablespoon chopped parsley

1. Sprinkle almonds with sugar and cook in a non-stick skillet over low heat, stirring until the sugar is melted and almonds are coated. Cool, break apart, and set aside.
2. Place cleaned greens in a plastic bag; add celery and onion; seal and refrigerate.
3. For the dressing: place all ingredients in a covered jar and shake well. Refrigerate.
5. Five minutes before serving, shake and pour dressing into the bag. Jiggle to cover the lettuce.
6. Pour into a serving bowl and dress with oranges and almonds.

6-8 servings

Notes

• *Use the prepared lettuce in bags to save time. Try a mix of spring greens and baby romaine. You could also add baby spinach and arugula for deep color and a little bite.*

• *If you don't want to fool with caramelizing the almonds, you can buy pre-sweetened almonds on the grocery store aisle with croutons and salad dressings. A great time-saver!*

• *Add a little freshly chopped parsley to the greens. Finish with a grind or two of fresh pepper.*

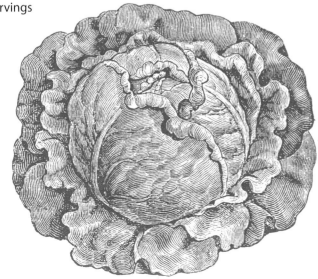

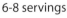

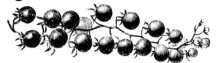

SALADS

Vegetable Salads

•LINDA DEAVER•

Strawberry Pecan Salad

Your favorite restaurant probably serves a version of this delicious salad. The combination of crisp greens, savory onions and blue cheese, and the sweet kick of fruit is a favorite at any gathering. Kids love the strawberries and pecans. If you are taking this to a potluck, carry the ingredients in separate containers and add together just before serving.

SALAD

Mixed greens
 (try red leaf because it is pretty with the strawberries)

Red onions, thinly sliced

Chopped pecans

Sliced strawberries

Blue cheese crumbles (optional)

DRESSING

1 cup sugar

1 cup vinegar

1 teaspoon dry mustard

1 cup canola oil

1 teaspoon salt

1 teaspoon paprika

3 cloves of garlic smashed
 or 1¹/₂ teaspoon crushed garlic (optional)

1. FOR THE DRESSING: place sugar & vinegar in saucepan over medium heat and stir occasionally until the sugar dissolves.
2. Mix in the mustard, oil, salt, and paprika; chill. If using garlic, add the smashed cloves to the mixture and leave until you are ready to add the dressing to the lettuce. Toss out the garlic and shake well to blend before you pour.
3. Fill a salad bowl with greens. Add the onions, strawberries, pecans and cheese, if using.
4. Toss gently with dressing just before serving.

Notes

• *If using blue cheese, you might want to try Maytag, since it is less creamy than Gorgonzola and crumbles a little better.*
• *Try substituting Parmesan cheese if timid palates are scared of blue cheese.*
• *Almonds work well in place of the pecans. Try a bag of the sugared almonds from the salad dressing aisle. Sugared pecans are also a nice variation.*
• *Figure on two cups of salad greens and filling per generous serving.*

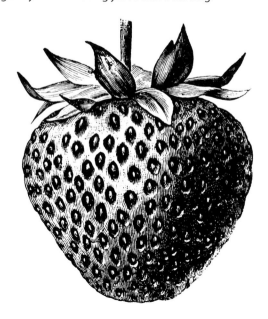

SALADS

Vegetable Salads

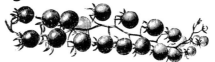

•WEBB FRIDAY NIGHT FEASTS•

Easy Caesar Salad

There may be fancier Caesar salads, but none easier than this one. Pre-washed bags of lettuce, bottled dressing and boxed croutons add up to a quick and easy dish. The high school boys always enjoyed it with just about any entrée. This is a great dish to assign to a working mom or dad who doesn't have much time for the kitchen for a class or team potluck.

4 heads of romaine lettuce, washed and dried or 2 bags of prewashed romaine

2 boxes onion and garlic croutons

1 cup shredded Parmesan cheese

2 bottles light Caesar dressing

Freshly ground black pepper

1. Place lettuce in a large serving bowl.
2. Just before serving, add salad dressing and toss thoroughly.
3. Finish with the cheese, croutons, and fresh pepper.

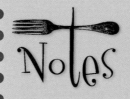

Notes

• When kids are serving themselves in a buffet line, use long tongs for dishing up salad rather than a fork and spoon serving set. You'll have less lettuce on the floor. The tongs can be used with one hand while the other one balances the plate.
• The quality of your Parmesan cheese makes a big difference in this recipe. Look for the pre-shredded cheese in the gourmet deli case; avoid anything in a can.
• Our favorite brands for this recipe were Pepperidge Farm Onion and Garlic Croutons and Giraud's light Caesar dressing.

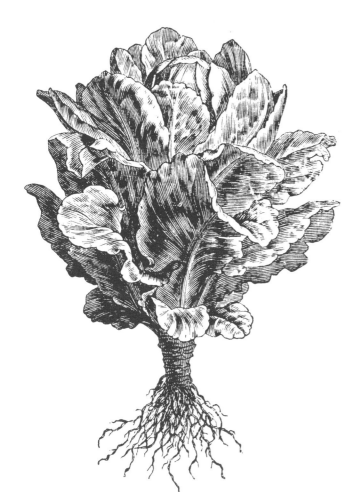

Vegetable Salads

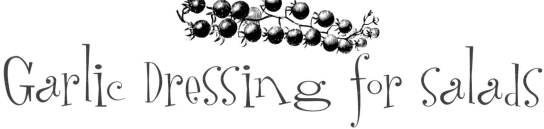

Garlic Dressing for Salads

This is a phenomenal dressing, full of garlic flavor without the bite. Cooking the garlic in water and oil mellows its flavor; the sugar and vinegar add a sweet/sour hit. This unusual dressing is perfect for a salad of greens and sliced vegetables. Be sure to finish it with some freshly shaved Parmesan cheese and cracked pepper.

10 large cloves of garlic, peeled and diced

1^1/$_4$ cups water

^{2}/$_3$ cups extra-virgin olive oil

^{1}/$_2$ teaspoon salt

Freshly ground black pepper

^{1}/$_2$ cup balsamic vinegar

^{1}/$_3$ cup red wine vinegar

2-3 tablespoons dark brown sugar

1. Combine the garlic, oil, water, salt and pepper in a skillet. Cover and simmer for 10 minutes, or until the garlic is soft. Pour into bowl and set aside.
2. Wipe out the skillet. Add the two vinegars and sugar. Bring to a boil and cook for 2 minutes. Taste for a sweet/sour balance. Really tart vinegar may need a bit more sugar for balance.
3. When you are ready to serve, combine the flavored oil with the vinegar mixture and bring to a soft boil. Spoon over the lettuce and finish with garnishes like cheese, nuts, onions and bacon.
4. About 2^1/$_2$ cups dressing

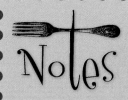

Notes

- *This dressing tastes especially good served with a salad that includes fresh herbs like basil, chives, parsley and oregano.*
- *Use a colorful mix of lettuces for a beautiful presentation. Try radicchio, arugula, romaine, butter lettuce and baby spinach.*
- *You could easily add chunks of meat or cheese to make this main dish salad. Salami or prosciutto would be perfect. Blue cheese would be heavenly.*

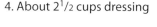

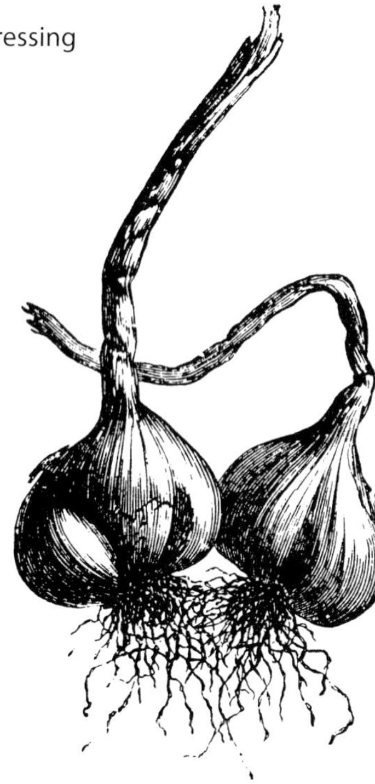

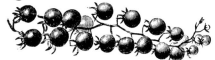

Vegetable Salads

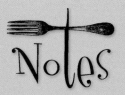

•LINDA DEAVER•

Bok Choy Salad

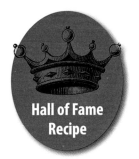

Hall of Fame Recipe

TRY THIS SALAD!!! It always gets rave reviews when I take it to a sick friend or potluck party. It sounds a little different, but it is a hit with young and old alike. The kids will be suckered in by the crunchy topping, and eat the vegetable part almost by accident. I like to keep some in the refrigerator for a quick snack or light meal. The bok choy is as mild as lettuce, but with more body. The sweet crunch of the topping paired with the smoothness of the bok choy and tang of the dressing make this dish fabulous.

$^1/_2$ **cup (1 stick) butter or margarine**

2 tablespoons sugar

1 cup sliced almonds

$^1/_2$ **cup (1 bottle) sesame seeds**

2   (3-ounce) packages of ramen noodles (crushed, remove seasoning packet)

1 bunch bok choy, green and white parts, thinly sliced

8 green onions, white and green parts, thinly sliced

DRESSING

$^3/_4$ **cup canola oil**

$^1/_2$ **cup red wine vinegar**

$^1/_3$ **cup sugar**

2 tablespoons soy sauce

1. Spray a skillet with non-stick spray. Melt the stick of butter and add the sugar. Stir until it dissolves.
2. Add the almonds, sesame seeds and ramen noodles, which have been crushed while still in the package. Try hitting the package with a rolling pin before opening to break up the noodles. Cook over medium heat, stirring constantly, until everything is well-coated with the butter. Watch closely, because the noodles can burn easily. Remove from heat when everything turns golden- this shouldn't take more than 10 minutes.
3. Cool and store the topping until ready to toss.
4. Combine dressing ingredients (oil, vinegar, sugar, soy sauce) in a small jar and shake to mix well.
5. When ready to serve, toss together the bok choy, onions, and noodle mixture in a large bowl (save a bit of the noodle mixture to garnish the top). Add the dressing a little at a time until all the bok choy is well coated, and toss thoroughly.

Notes

• *This makes a whole lot of noodle topping. You could easily double the amount of bok choy in the recipe and still have plenty of noodles and dressing to go around. If I use just one bunch of bok choy, I use only half the noodles*

•*I never use all the dressing in one sitting. It will keep for another round or two of salad in a few days. You will probably still have some noodle mixture left over, too.*

• *Bok Choy is really the best green for this the recipe, although other lettuces would be delicious, too. It has a lovely, mild flavor and the leaves have a velvety texture. Use the crisper, white part of the stem, too – it is mild and crunchy. It also adds texture and color contrast. It really is shocking that something so good for you actually tastes great.*

• *The plain salad is delicious – but you can add so much to make it really spectacular. Try a little chopped red or yellow bell pepper and some bright red sliced radishes for color. Fresh herbs like oregano, cilantro, parsley or basil brighten the flavor, while the addition of tangy arugula lettuce makes a nice contrast to the milder bok choy. Diced cucumber, carrot rounds, chopped celery – all would be wonderful additions. I would not add tomatoes, however. Their flavor and texture competes with the noodle topping.*

• *If you want to lower the fat, use less butter for the noodle sauté. The full dose is yummy, but you really need just enough butter to coat the ingredients and brown them. Cut the portion down to half a stick, and test for taste and texture. Or, start with 2 tablespoons and see if you like the result – you can always add more.*

Vegetable Salads

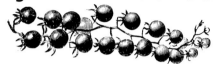

•PAM MULLINS•

Ramen Noodle Salad

This is a popular salad that is perfect for a buffet. Everyone loves the crunchy sweet and tart flavors. The packaged broccoli slaw makes it quick and easy to make. Prepare it a few days ahead and let it mature in the fridge – it only gets better. Older kids like this salad.

2 packages Ramen chicken noodles, crushed

2 packages Broccoli Slaw

$^1/_2$ cup green onions, sliced

$^1/_2$ cup sliced almonds

1 cup plain (not roasted) sunflower seeds

DRESSING

$^1/_3$ cup sugar

$^2/_3$ cup cider vinegar

Seasoning from noodle package

$^1/_2$ cup good quality olive oil

1. Before opening the ramen noodles, hit the package several times with a rolling pin or other heavy utensil to break up the noodles.
2. Combine the ingredients for the dressing in a jar and shake well to blend.
3. Toss all the salad ingredients together in a bowl and add the dressing. Mix well to ensure everything is blended. Refrigerate until ready to use.

Serves 8

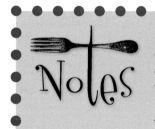

Notes
• *You can use sweet Vidalia onions when they are in season instead of the green onions.*
• *Feel free to add other vegetables to the mix: chopped peppers, sliced carrots, cucumbers.*

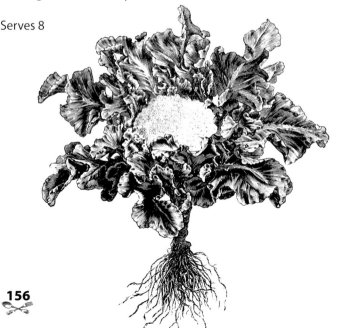

RAMEN SALAD SIDEBAR

These two salads are similar in that they both use ramen noodles and a sweet/sour dressing. But they taste very different. The first one cooks the noodles in butter along with the almonds, creating a cooked, crispy topping. The second salad uses raw ingredients that benefit from a 24-hour marinade. It also uses the seasoning packet from the ramen noodles that adds a savory layer of flavor. They are both delicious – and popular! – side dishes at a potluck. Don't be afraid of the bok choy in the first recipe – it is very mildly flavored and has a lovely velvety texture.

Vegetable Salads

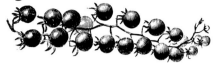

•DIANE ROBBINS•

Spaghetti Salad

This one has to be made ahead, and the longer it sits, the better it gets. It is sort of like potato salad with pasta instead. A lemony vinaigrette and crunchy vegetables work beautifully with the pasta – people find it difficult to quit eating this stuff! It is the ultimate buffet dish and nice to have on hand when there are lots of hungry teenagers in the house.

MARINADE:

1 tablespoon Accent

1 tablespoon Lawry's seasoned salt

4 tablespoons olive oil

3 tablespoons fresh lemon juice

SALAD:

16 ounces vermicelli, cooked and drained

1 small jar diced pimentos

1 cup chopped green pepper

$^3/_4$ cup chopped onion

1 small can chopped black olives

2 cups diced celery

$^1/_2$ cup mayonnaise

1. Combine the ingredients for the marinade and pour over the cooked pasta. Toss until the noodles are well-coated. Refrigerate overnight.
2. The next day, add the pimentos, green pepper, onion, olives, celery, and mayonnaise. Toss well to disperse the vegetables through the pasta. Let the salad sit several hours before serving.

Serves 8-10 generously

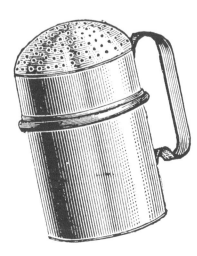

Notes

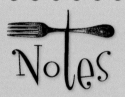

• For the overnight step, I like to mix the marinade in a zip-top bag, throw in the cooked pasta and move it all around until the pasta is covered.

• I find it is easier to toss the mayonnaise and vegetables in with the pasta if I use a large roasting pan instead of a bowl. I can spread everything out in a thin layer and make sure there are no clumps of pasta that don't get covered with dressing. After combining the ingredients, I store the salad in a large bowl.

• This salad improves with time. Make it ahead several days.

• This recipe is a hit in the summer time, great if you are serving house guests.

• This is an easy one to spruce up. Try adding roasted veggies, avocado and bacon, or boiled shrimp. Chopped fresh herbs would be good, too, especially parsley. Use $^1/_4$ - $^1/_2$ cup.

• Try using Kalamata olives from the deli department instead of the canned olives.

• If you don't want the onion in this dish to be too assertive, soak it in ice water for about $^1/_2$ hour before adding. Or use $^1/_2$ teaspoon onion powder instead of the onion.

Vegetable Salads

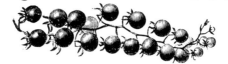

•SUSAN PORTER LEVY•

Mediterranean Couscous Salad

Susan is an accomplished cook with a terrific nose for good recipes. She is also very good about preparing healthy food for her family. This is one of their favorite recipes. It is savory and fresh tasting with all the parsley and vegetables. Teenagers like this one. It is a good vegetarian offering.

1 box couscous mix

One dozen cherry tomatoes (quartered)

One cucumber, peeled, seeded, diced

4 ounces Feta cheese, diced

1 cup parsley, chopped

Bottled Greek vinaigrette salad dressing.

Fresh lemon (optional)

1. Prepare couscous according to the directions on the box. Cool the mixture.
2. Add the tomatoes, cucumbers, Feta and parsley to the couscous and dress with the Greek vinaigrette. Taste for seasoning. Drizzle the juice from a fresh lemon half over the mixture, if desired.
3. Chill for at least several hours. Toss well before serving.

Serves 6-8

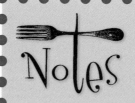

Notes

• *Susan likes to use the roasted garlic and olive oil flavored couscous for this recipe. There are a number of delicious variations – experiment!*
• *And speaking of olives, why not toss in a few spicy ripe olives?*
• *Another great addition would be a little fresh mint, chopped fine.*
• *If using this for a vegetarian dish, add a little extra cheese for the protein.*

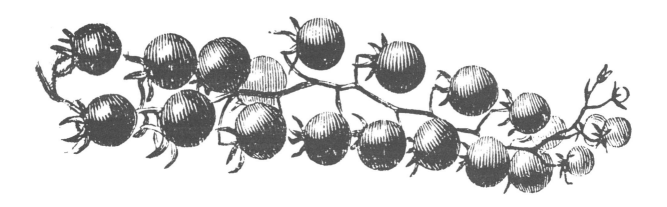

Entrée Salads

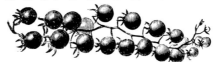

•CINDY BAIRD•

Mom's Chicken Salad

This is a wonderful, old-fashioned recipe with a sweet addition of pineapple and nuts. It avoids mayonnaise, using cream cheese and sour cream instead. This would be lovely served in lettuce cups with a small bowl of soup and cheese toast (cheese toast makes everything better!) Save this one for the adults.

3-ounce package of cream cheese, warmed to room temperature

$^1/_2$ cup sour cream

$^3/_4$ cup celery

$^1/_2$ cup walnuts

2 tablespoons chopped green pepper

1$^1/_2$ cups cooked chicken

1 13-ounce can Dole pineapple tidbits, drained

Salt to taste

1. Mix the sour cream and cream cheese until well-blended.
2. Carefully stir in the remaining ingredients. Chill until ready to serve.

Serves 4-6

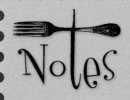 **Notes**

• *If you need to loosen the mixture, add a little extra sour cream or some half and half.*
• *Boiled chicken makes the mildest, most delicate-tasting salad. You could also use roasted chicken, which has a stronger flavor, if that is what you have on hand. Or pick up a pre-cooked chicken at the grocery for even less effort.*
• *Fresh pineapple would be wonderful in this salad. Since its texture is firmer, try cutting it a little smaller than the tidbits that come in a can.*

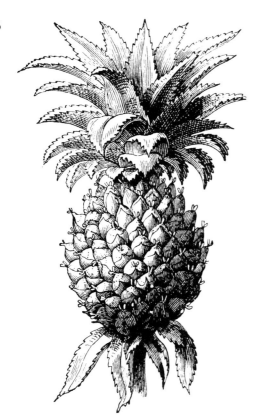

SALADS

Entrée Salads

•HELEN GEORGI•

shrimp salad

This recipe comes to me from a dear friend of my mother who always served the most elegant ladies' lunches. Don't be fooled by the short ingredient list. This is a rich salad, full of flavor. Save it for a special occasion and let it be the star of the menu, accompanied by cheese toast and a fruit plate.

5 pounds of shrimp (31-35 count), boiled, peeled, deveined, and loosely chopped

1 cup dill pickle relish

2 cups finely chopped celery

1$^1/_2$ - 2 cups mayonnaise

1 teaspoon hot sauce

2 tablespoons Worcestershire sauce

Tomato, lemon wedge for garnish

1. Combine all ingredients except shrimp, using 1$^1/_2$ cups mayonnaise. Mix well.
2. Fold in shrimp. Add more mayonnaise if the mixture seems dry. Refrigerate.
3. Serve on lettuce beds with wedges of tomato and lemon.

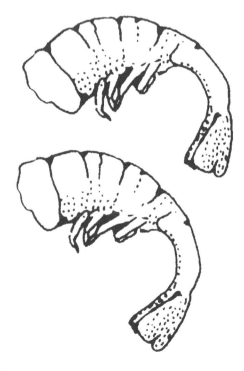

Notes

• *The sauce can be made a day or two ahead and the shrimp can be cooked ahead, too. Keep separate until you are ready to serve. Fold the cooked shrimp into the sauce at the last minute.*

• *To keep the texture of the shrimp from becoming mushy when boiling, try this technique from Cook's Illustrated test kitchen: In a large pot, combine 5-6 cups cold water with the juice from 2 lemons and the spent halves, a tablespoon each of salt and sugar, a handful of whole peppercorns and a grind of fresh pepper, and one bunch of parsley. Add the shrimp to the pot of cold water and place over medium heat. Cook until the shrimp turn pink, at least 15 minutes. The water will not come to a boil (it should read 165 degrees on an instant thermometer and just begin bubbling). Remove the pot and cover. Let the shrimp sit for 2 minutes. Drain and plunge into a large bowl of ice water to stop the cooking. I always test one shrimp before I drain them, just in case they need another minute or two of steeping. This cold start and steam bath finish produce a nice, non-rubbery or mushy shrimp.*

Entrée Salads

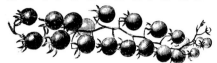

•SUSAN PORTER LEVY•

Shrimp Salad With Black Bean Salsa

This easy, easy shrimp salad has all the flavors of Susan's Dallas hometown: beans and corn, salsa and cilantro. This is a great "quick fix" for a weeknight dinner, but has real potential at a ladies' lunch. It would make an impressive addition to a tailgate, served over a bowl of ice to keep the shrimp happy. If you use it at a buffet, just chop up the avocado and throw it (carefully!) in with the salad.

1¹/₂ pounds medium shrimp, peeled and deveined

1 tablespoon butter

¹/₄ teaspoon roasted garlic powder

2 tablespoons fresh lime juice

1¹/₂ cups frozen whole kernel corn, thawed

³/₄ jar chipotle salsa (Frontera brand preferred)

1 15-ounce can black beans, rinsed and drained

¹/₄ cup chopped fresh cilantro

Avocado slices

1. Melt butter in large saucepan, add garlic powder. When butter is just beginning to brown, add shrimp and cook until done. Add lime juice. Remove from heat.
2. Stir in corn, salsa, and beans. Place in bowl and toss with cilantro. Cover and refrigerate.
3. Serve cold over lettuce leaves with slices of avocado spritzed with lime juice.

Serves 4-6

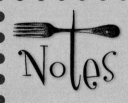

Notes

• *For a different sort of garlic flavor, throw in a little mashed garlic with the butter before you sauté the shrimp. You could still use the garlic powder.*
• *If the salsa doesn't add enough kick for you, a sprinkle of cayenne would.*

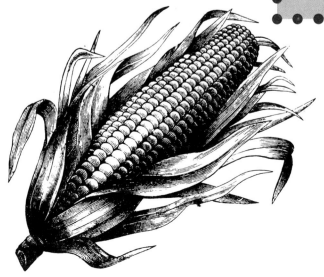

RECIPES

DESSERT

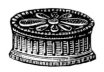
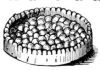

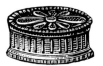

Cakes and Cookies

Best Cake Mix

A friend shared this variation on cake mix a number of years ago. It makes the lightest, moistest cake – it takes any mix and elevates it to the "I HAVE to have that recipe!" category. People will be surprised to learn it all started with a box! Just ignore the directions and ingredients on the back of the box and use this instead. Use any mix or brand.

1 box cake mix
1 egg
1 egg white
1^1/$_3$ cup water
^{1}/$_2$ stick unsalted butter (4 tablespoons), room temp

1. Preheat the oven to 300 degrees.
2. Prepare two cake pans with non-stick spray.
3. Combine all ingredients.
4. Bake for 40 minutes.

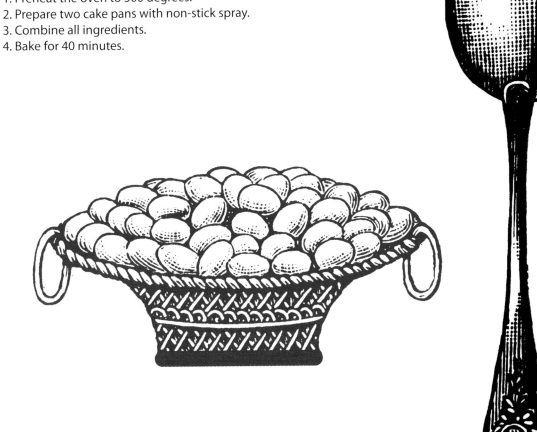

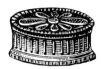

•SHIRLEY JARVIS•

Chocolate Wax Cake

This is the all-time favorite for birthdays and get-togethers in the Jarvis family. It combines moist chocolate cake with caramel frosting. Perfect!

CAKE:

3 cups plain flour

2 cups white sugar

4 heaping tablespoons cocoa

1 teaspoon salt

2 teaspoon soda

$^1/_2$ cup + 2 tablespoons canola oil

2 cups water

2 tablespoons vinegar

2 teaspoons vanilla

1. Preheat the oven to 360 degrees (325 for a glass pan.) Grease and flour a 9x13-inch pan.
2. In a large bowl, sift together the dry ingredients (flour, sugar, cocoa, salt and soda.)
3. Add the oil, water, vinegar and vanilla; beat until smooth.
4. Bake for 35-40 minutes. Test for doneness at 35 minutes. Do NOT overbake. This cake is very moist and waxy.
5. Cool and frost with one of the Caramel Frostings, recipes below.

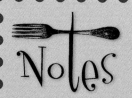

Notes

- *Take the time to grease and flour the cake pan; non-stick spray won't do the job.*
- *The first caramel icing is tricky to prepare, but it is Shirley's favorite topping for this favorite cake. It has a delicious praline taste and unique texture. The first time you try it, have the ingredients for the other icing on hand as a back-up. If you cook the syrup too long, it will harden like candy - you won't be spreading it on any cake! But it will make a tasty confection that could be dipped in chocolate or crumbled over ice cream. Or eaten right out of the pan once it cools!*
- *A thermometer is the best way to determine when the syrup reaches the soft ball stage, since weather can affect the way the syrup balls up in water.*

"OLD TIMEY" CARAMEL FROSTING:

1 stick ($^1/_2$ cup) butter

2 cups light brown sugar, packed

$^1/_2$ cup Carnation evaporated milk

(reserve extra from a small can for adding

while beating, if necessary)

1. Combine all ingredients in a sauce pan. Bring to a boil, stirring constantly. Cook to soft ball stage (234-240 degrees) or until a few drops form a soft ball when dropped in very cold water.
2. Place the pan in cold water and beat the syrup until it thickens to spreading consistency.

EASY CARAMEL FROSTING:

1 stick ($^1/_2$ cup) butter, melted

1 cup brown sugar, packed

$^1/_4$ cup milk

$1^1/_2$ - 2 cups sifted powdered sugar

1. In a saucepan, add sugar to melted butter and bring to a boil. Boil 2 minutes.
2. Add milk and bring back to a boil then remove from heat.
3. Cool a few minutes and slowly add the sifted powdered sugar.

DESSERT

Cakes and Cookies

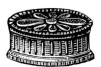

• SHIRLEY JARVIS •

Texas Sheet Cake

This recipe has appeared in nearly every cookbook since Gutenberg invented the printing press. And for good reason – this is a perennial favorite with the kids, their parents, and visiting relatives. Need a dessert for a school event that won't leave you with any leftovers? This is it.

CAKE:

2 cups flour

2 cups sugar

$^1/_2$ cup (1 stick) butter

$^1/_2$ cup shortening

1 cup water

3 tablespoons cocoa

2 eggs, slightly beaten

$^1/_2$ cup buttermilk

1 teaspoon baking soda

2 teaspoons vanilla

ICING:

$^1/_2$ cup butter

3 tablespoons cocoa powder (Dutch is best)

6 tablespoons milk

1 1-pound box powdered sugar (3$^1/_2$ - 4 cups)

2 teaspoons vanilla extract

1. Bring the butter, cocoa and milk to a boil.
2. Remove from the heat and add the sugar and vanilla. Beat until thoroughly mixed.

1. Preheat the oven to 350 degrees. Grease an 11x15-inch pan.
2. Combine the flour and sugar in a large bowl and set aside.
3. In a sauce pan, combine the butter, shortening, water and cocoa. Bring to a boil.
4. Pour the mixture over the flour and sugar; mix well.
5. Add the eggs, buttermilk, soda and vanilla.
6. Mix well and pour into a greased, 11x15 pan.
7. Bake for 25 minutes at 350 degrees. Remove from the oven and pour icing over the hot cake. Let the iced cake cool, and then cut into squares for serving.

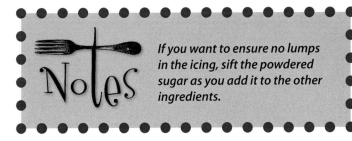

Notes

If you want to ensure no lumps in the icing, sift the powdered sugar as you add it to the other ingredients.

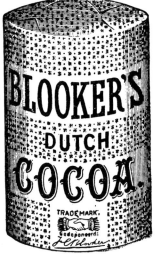

BLOOKER'S DUTCH COCOA.

TRADE MARK.

Cakes and Cookies

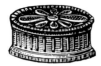

•DIANE ROBBINS•

Three-day Coconut Cake

This is the perfect holiday or event recipe. It must be made three days in advance and the cake just gets better as it sits. Don't skip the step dividing the layers in half –it is one of the secrets to this cake's success. The thin layers of cake are permeated with the sour cream/coconut mixture as it sits, and each bite is gooey-moist, full of coconut flavor.

One box yellow butter cake mix

1³/₄ cups sugar

1 16-ounce container (2 cups) sour cream

12 ounces shredded coconut - frozen is best

9 ounce container of frozen topping (Cool Whip preferred)

1. Prepare the cake mix according to package directions, making two layers.
2. When completely cool, slice each layer in half horizontally with a serrated knife. This makes a four-layer cake.
3. Combine sugar, sour cream and coconut, blending well. Let this mixture set for 30 minutes in the refrigerator.
4. Reserve 1 cup sour cream mixture for topping. Spread the remainder between layers of cake.
5. Combine reserved sour cream mixture with Cool Whip; blend until smooth. Spread on top and sides of cake. Seal the cake in an airtight container, or wrap the cake plate securely with plastic wrap. REFRIGERATE FOR THREE (3) DAYS BEFORE SERVING.
6. Set the cake out at least 30 minutes before serving; if any cake is left over, keep in the refrigerator.

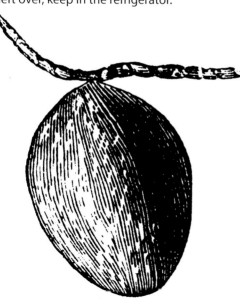

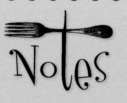

Notes

• *Try adding a teaspoon of vanilla or almond flavoring to the cake mix. Or try varying the flavor of the cake mix you use. I have had delicious results with lemon, butter, even orange mixes. I have never tried chocolate, but I think it just might be fabulous. You can use the mixes that have pudding in them for an even moister result.*

• *You can use sweetened, bagged coconut instead of frozen, but you will have a much sweeter finished product.*

• *Slicing the cake layers in half can be tricky; be sure to use a knife long enough to go all the way through the entire circumference of the layer.*

• *You can save some coconut to toast and sprinkle on the top. Spread coconut out on a flat, microwave-safe dish. Cook in 30 second intervals, stirring after each interval, until the coconut is a golden toasty color. Do not toast all the coconut used in the recipe – only for the garnish on top.*

• *If you are serving this cake for Easter or a color-themed event, you can dye your coconut with a little food coloring. Again, this would be some extra coconut you sprinkle on top for a finishing garnish. Pastels are lovely for a spring event, and a two-color team theme would be fun for a sporting event.*

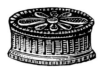

DESSERT

Cakes and Cookies

•DIANE ROBBINS•

Coconut Cake

This recipe has been around for a long time and has never lessened in popularity. It is a "must-have" at Diane's house during the Christmas holidays. It is an easy one to make, and so darn good –gooey and coconut-y. As the cake sits in the fridge, it just gets moister and moister, though it never gets much of a chance to really develop that moisture at my house. Gone too soon.

1 box of yellow butter cake mix

1 stick of butter, softened

5 eggs, separated

$^1/_2$ cup water

1 can Eagle brand sweetened condensed milk

1 15-ounce can cream of coconut (Coco Lopez preferred)

1 large container frozen whipped topping

1-2 packages frozen coconut, thawed

1. Preheat the oven to 350 degrees. Grease and flour a 12x18-inch pan. Don't use non-stick spray; take the time to grease and flour.
2. Mix together cake mix, butter, egg yolks and water.
3. Beat the egg whites until stiff, but not dry, and fold carefully into the cake mixture.
4. Bake in prepared pan for 20 minutes.
5. While the cake is baking, mix together the condensed milk and cream of coconut.
6. Remove the cake from the oven and while it is hot, punch holes in the surface with a toothpick. Pour the coconut/milk mixture over the top. When the cake is completely cooled, cover with the whipped topping and sprinkle with the coconut. Refrigerate.

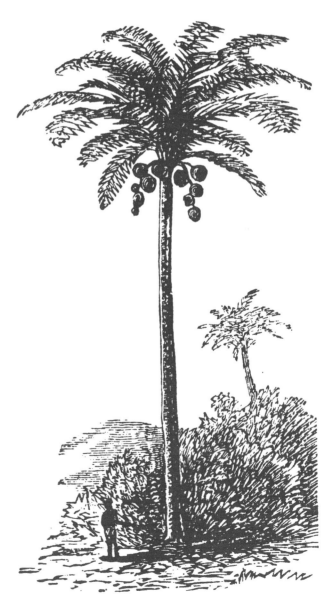

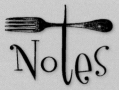 Notes

• *Try different flavors of cake mixes – lemon and plain white are delicious, too! I have never tried chocolate, but I'm thinking it would work.*
• *You can use freshly whipped cream instead of frozen topping for a rich variation. Or try light frozen whipped topping to save a smidge of calories. Seems pointless, considering the rest of the ingredients, though. . .*

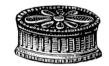

Cakes and Cookies

•KATHY HALL•

Fresh Apple Spice Cake

This cake is a moist treat. The butterscotch chips eliminate the need for icing, so it is less messy to eat than some other cakes. You will definitely need napkins because it is so lusciously moist. Be sure to take the cake out of the pan after a short cooling, otherwise it will cling and tear when you try to remove it. If you are making this for kids, you could leave out the nuts.

2 cups sugar

2 eggs

1 cup oil

$^1/_2$ cup water

2 teaspoons baking powder

1 teaspoon soda

2$^1/_2$ cups flour

1 teaspoon salt

1 teaspoon cinnamon

2$^1/_2$ cups diced apples

1 cup chopped nuts, pecans or walnuts (optional)

1 12-ounce package butterscotch morsels

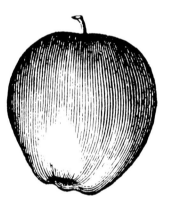

1. Preheat oven to 350 degrees. Grease and flour a 13x9x2-inch baking pan. Do not use non-stick spray.
2. Mix together the sugar, eggs, water and oil.
3. In another bowl, combine the baking powder, soda, flour, salt and cinnamon.
4. Combine the apples and nuts in a bowl.
5. Add the dry ingredients to the wet mixture, alternating with the apples / nut mixture. Begin and end with the dry ingredients. You will add about a third of the flour, mix well, and then stir in half the apples and nuts. Repeat, adding a third of the flour, mixing well and stirring in the remaining fruit and nuts. End with the flour and mix well.
6. Pour the batter into the prepared pan and sprinkle with the butterscotch morsels. Bake for 1 hour.
7. Cool and cut into small squares. Use a spatula to remove squares from the pan. The cake is very moist on the bottom and wants to stick. Don't let it!

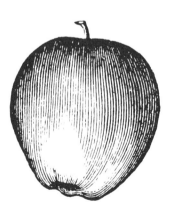

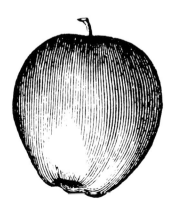

DESSERT

Cakes and Cookies

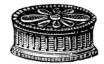

•LEAH MOIR•

Ice Cream Sandwich Cake

Simple, simple, simple. The hardest part of this recipe is unwrapping the ice cream sandwiches. This is a hit with the kids every time. To serve at a buffet, use a cooler until you are ready to serve.

1 box of ice cream sandwiches

1 jar caramel ice cream sauce

1 small container of whipped topping

I bag of crushed candy bars like Heath or Skor

1. Fill a large pan with a layer of half the ice cream sandwiches.
2. Drizzle liberally with caramel sauce and stack on remaining sandwiches.
3. Drizzle again with the caramel sauce.
4. Cover the surface with whipped topping and sprinkle with a generous layer of crushed candy bar. Freeze.

Serves 12

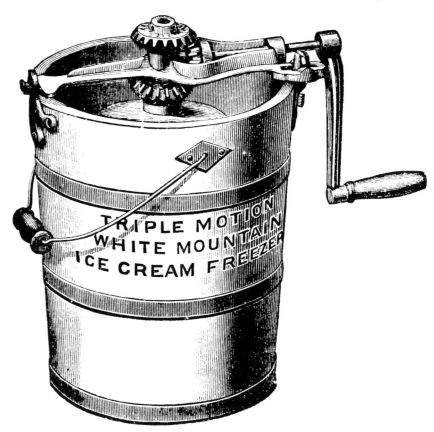

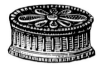
•JOAN JORDAN•

Pistachio Cake

Do you want to make your reputation at the next tailgate or church potluck? Take this cake, and be prepared to share the recipe. The texture of this cake is incredibly moist and light. It goes together in under ten minutes and I'll bet you'll want to eat it all at one sitting after you taste the first bite.

1 package white cake mix (Betty Crocker brand preferred)

1 package instant pistachio pudding mix

$^1/_2$ cup water

$^1/_2$ cup vegetable oil

$^1/_2$ cup orange juice

4 eggs

$^2/_3$ cup Hershey's chocolate syrup

1. Preheat the oven to 350 degrees. Grease and flour a bundt pan or a 9x13-inch pan.
2. Mix all ingredients together except the chocolate syrup and beat for 5 minutes. Be sure to beat the entire 5 minutes.
3. Take 3/4 of the batter and pour into the bundt pan. Mix the Hershey's chocolate syrup with the remaining batter and pour on top.
4. Bake for 35 - 50 minutes until done. Be careful not to over cook! Start checking for doneness after 35 minutes. A bundt cake will take longer than one cooked in the flat pan.
5. Cool for ten minutes then remove from pan. Cover tightly. This keeps the cake very moist.

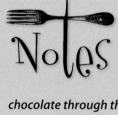

Notes

• *To ensure a clean release, take the time to butter and flour the bundt pan.*
• *If you prefer to have the chocolate run through the cake rather than sit on top, swirl the chocolate through the batter before baking.*
• *You can use an angel food bundt pan.*
• *Try serving this with freshly whipped cream, a sprinkling of shaved chocolate, and salted (shelled!) pistachios. Or drizzle some chocolate syrup over it for a messy treat.*
• *Kids don't need to hear the word "pistachio" associated with this cake. It might spook 'em. Focus on the chocolate.*

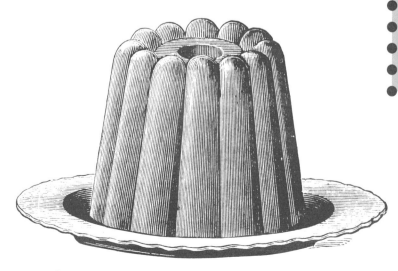

Cakes and Cookies

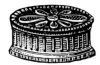

•SHIRLEY JARVIS•

Rum Fruit Cake

This is a favorite holiday dessert in Shirley's family. It looks difficult, with lots of ingredients, but is actually easy. It is completely different from traditional, hard-as-a-brick fruitcakes from days of yore. This one uses fresh apples and bananas, some chopped nuts and a bit of rum and spices for flavoring. The glaze is sweetened, rum-infused apple juice. This would be great on a holiday buffet menu and the ultimate homemade Christmas gift.

CAKE:

3 eggs

1 cup white sugar

1 cup brown sugar, lightly packed

1 teaspoon vanilla

3 cups plain flour

$^1/_2$ teaspoon salt

2 teaspoons baking soda

1 teaspoon cinnamon

$^1/_2$ teaspoon nutmeg

$^1/_2$ teaspoon ground cloves

$1^1/_2$ cup canola oil

2 cups raw chopped apples

2 cups chopped bananas

$^1/_2$ cup chopped dates

1 cup chopped pecans

$^1/_4$ cup light rum

Glaze:

$^1/_3$ cup apple juice

$^1/_4$ cup rum

2 cups powdered sugar

1. Preheat oven to 350 degrees. Grease and flour a bundt pan.
2. Prepare fruits and set aside.
3. Beat eggs in a mixer on medium speed until lemon-colored, about five minutes. Add white and brown sugar and vanilla. Blend.
4. In another bowl, mix together the flour, salt, baking soda, cinnamon, nutmeg and cloves.
5. Beginning and ending with dry ingredients, alternately add dry mixture and oil to the egg mixture, incorporating the flour well after each addition.
6. Fold in the fruit and nuts; add rum and mix well. Pour into prepared pan.
7. Bake for one hour.
8. As soon as the cake comes out of the oven, loosen the sides and center around the tube with a thin knife.
9. Combine the glaze ingredients and slowly spoon over the cake and around the sides and tube. Let stand 5 minutes before removing from the pan.

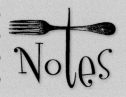

Notes

• *Go to the extra trouble of greasing and flouring the cake pan; non-stick spray will not do the job.*

• *For even more flavor, toast the pecans before using them. Heat nuts in a skillet over medium high heat for about five minutes. Watch carefully to prevent burning.*

• *This cake ages well. It is even better after several days in a cool, unheated room.*

• *The rum glaze may ooze; wrap completely to catch any overrun.*

• *Leftovers freeze well.*

• *Serve with whipped cream or boiled custard.*

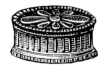

•SHIRLEY JARVIS•

Upside Down German Chocolate Cake

This cake is easy to prepare – especially since it doesn't need to be frosted. Once you get it in the oven, the job is over! The dollops of sweetened cream cheese spread throughout the cake are a moist surprise; you get the creamy texture mixed in with the cake texture without the mess of icing. And of course, you have all those pecans and coconut. This is a great one for the buffet line.

1 cup coconut

1 cup chopped pecans

1 box of German chocolate cake mix

8 ounces cream cheese, softened

1 box powdered sugar

1 stick butter, melted

1 teaspoon vanilla

1. Preheat the oven to 350 degrees. Prepare a 9x13-inch pan by buttering it and coating with flour. This will give a better release than non-stick spray.
2. Layer the coconut and nuts in the prepared pan.
3. Mix the cake according to the directions on the box and pour over the nuts and coconut.
4. Stir together the cream cheese, powdered sugar, butter, and vanilla; spread or dollop over the cake batter.
5. Bake at 350 degrees for 45 minutes. It will look gooey after it is done.

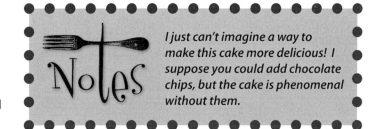

Notes

I just can't imagine a way to make this cake more delicious! I suppose you could add chocolate chips, but the cake is phenomenal without them.

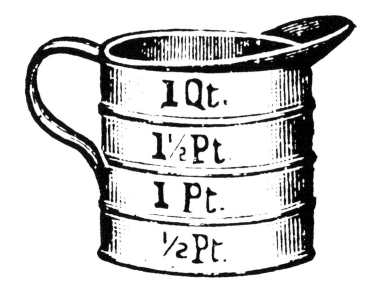

1 Qt.

1½ Pt

1 Pt.

½ Pt.

Cakes and Cookies

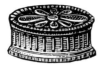

·CINDY BAIRD·

Creamy New York Cheesecake

Cheesecake is a kid-favorite. Even the calorie-conscious girls make room for a bite or two of this fabulous dessert. This recipe is one of the richest, most decadent I've seen, using five instead of the normal three packages of cream cheese. Pair this with a simple entrée, since you don't want to kill your crowd with too much rich food. This could be topped with fresh fruit to dilute the impact.

CRUST:

$^3/_4$ **cup all purpose flour**

6 tablespoons butter, softened

3 tablespoons sugar

$^1/_2$ **tablespoon vanilla**

1 egg yolk

FILLING:

5 8-ounce packages cream cheese, softened

3 tablespoons self-rising flour

1$^3/_4$ cups sugar

5 tablespoons lemon juice

3 tablespoons vanilla

5 eggs

2 egg yolks

TOPPING:

8 ounces sour cream

$^1/_2$ **cup sugar**

1 teaspoon vanilla

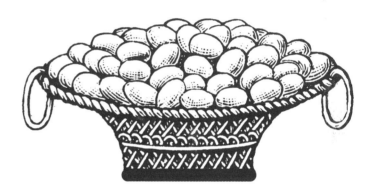

FOR THE CRUST:

1. Preheat the oven to 300 degrees. Lightly grease spring-form pan.
2. Mix all ingredients for the crust together in the bowl of a food processor. Pulse a few times until blended.
3. Spread $^1/_2$ of crust mix on bottom of pan, leaving off the side portion. Bake at 300 for 5 minutes.
4. Spread remaining crust mix around the sides of the pan.

FOR THE FILLING:

1. Preheat the oven to 500 degrees. Cream the softened cream cheese one package at a time in a very large mixing bowl.
2. Add flour and sugar and mix well. Beat in lemon juice and vanilla. Beat in eggs and yolks.
3. Pour in spring form pan. Bake at 500 degrees for 12 minutes. Reduce to 200 degrees and bake 50 - 60 minutes.
4. For the topping: While the filling is cooking, beat together sour cream, sugar, and vanilla.
5. Pour over top of cheesecake after it comes out of the oven and bake 10 more minutes at 350 degrees.

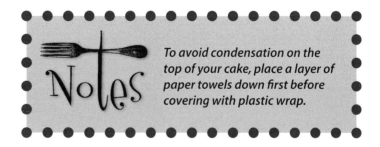

Notes

To avoid condensation on the top of your cake, place a layer of paper towels down first before covering with plastic wrap.

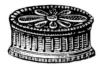

Cakes and Cookies

•MAUREEN ROWAN•

Congo Brownies

Maureen baked cookies professionally and she is not only a great baker, but a perfectionist in the kitchen as well. This is her favorite blond brownie recipe. The chocolate chips make if almost like a giant, moist, thick chocolate chip cookie. Like a pound cake, it has few ingredients, so the flavors are pure and satisfying. Kids love these. So do parents.

- **1^1/$_2$ sticks (^{3}/$_4$ cups) butter**
- **1 pound (1 box) dark brown sugar**
- **3 eggs, beaten**
- **2^3/$_4$ cups flour**
- **1^1/$_2$ teaspoon baking powder**
- **^{1}/$_2$ teaspoon salt**
- **12-ounce package of chocolate chips**
- **1 cup chopped pecans**

1. Preheat the oven to 350 degrees. Lightly grease and flour a 9x13-inch pan.
2. Melt the butter and then pour over the brown sugar in a large mixing bowl.
3. Add the beaten eggs to the butter and sugar, then mix well.
4. In another bowl, combine the flour, baking powder and salt and mix well. Slowly add the mixture to the butter mixture.
5. Add the chips and nuts, mixing carefully by hand to incorporate. Pour into the prepared pan.
6. Bake for 35 minutes. Do not over-bake. Cut into squares.

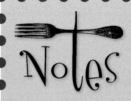

Notes

- *To make sure I don't get any lumps of baking powder or salt, I like to do my own version of sifting dry ingredients: I hold a medium-holed strainer over a bowl and dump in the dry ingredients. A few shakes and all the ingredients pass through the strainer and blend. Now they are ready to add to the wet ingredients.*
- *As always, toasted pecans add a depth of flavor. Toss the raw pecans into a skillet over medium heat and cook about 5 minutes, stirring and never leaving the pan since the nuts will easily burn.*

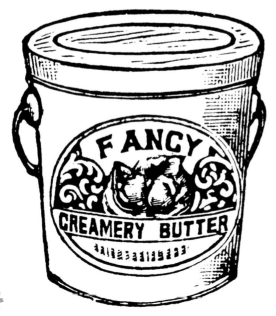

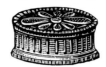

Cakes and Cookies

·JOAN JORDAN·

chocolate chip treasure cookies

Wow, are these good! And so easy to make. They are a nice change from the standard chocolate chip cookie: crunchy from the cracker crumbs, and gooey-moist from the condensed milk. You could leave out the coconut or nuts if you are dealing with kids who have allergies, and still have a wonderful concoction.

1^1/$_2$ **cups graham cracker crumbs**

^{1}/$_2$ **cup all-purpose flour**

2 teaspoons baking powder

1 14-ounce can Eagle Brand Condensed Milk (sweetened)

^{1}/$_2$ **cup margarine or butter, softened (1 stick)**

1 3^1/$_2$-ounce can flaked coconut (1^1/$_2$ cups)

1 12-ounce package semi-sweet chocolate chips (2 cups)

1 cup chopped walnuts

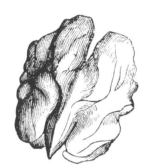

1. Heat oven to 375 degrees. Spray cookie sheet with non-stick spray.
2. In small bowl, mix graham cracker crumbs, flour and baking powder.
3. In larger mixer bowl, beat sweetened condensed milk and margarine until smooth. Add graham cracker crumb mixture; hand mix well. Stir in coconut, chocolate chips and walnuts.
4. Drop by rounded teaspoon onto ungreased cookie sheet.
5. Bake 9 to 10 minutes or until lightly browned.
6. Store loosely covered at room temperature.

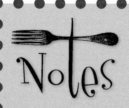

Notes

• *This is a wonderful basic recipe that can be expanded and adapted. Start experimenting with the last three ingredients.*
• *Instead of chocolate chips, you could use toffee chips or any other bagged candy bits from the baking aisle.*
• *You could use different nuts, like pecans, peanuts or cashews.*
• *Instead of coconut, you could add an equal amount of pretzels, smushed into large pieces, and some M&M's instead of chocolate chips, and skip the nuts.*
• *Maybe peanuts and raisins instead of coconut and walnuts? You get the idea. Suit the season or the audience with substitutions. Play around.*

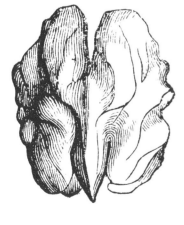

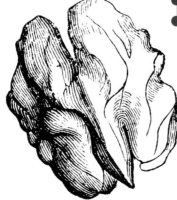

Cakes and Cookies

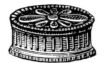

•PATTI PEARSON•

Enhanced Chocolate Chip Cookies

These are a variation on the basic Toll House cookie recipe on the back of every package of chocolate chips. It makes a huge, rich, chewy cookie that kids adore. It is a cookie on steroids. They are a great finish to a meal for kids or teenagers.

1 recipe Toll House cookies
1 cup chocolate chips

1. Make the cookie dough according to instructions on the back of the chocolate chip bag. Add the extra cup of chocolate chips.
2. Form the dough into balls and refrigerate about 2 hours (but more is OK).
3. Cook at 365 degrees instead of 375 degrees for only 7-9 minutes. Cool on a wire rack.

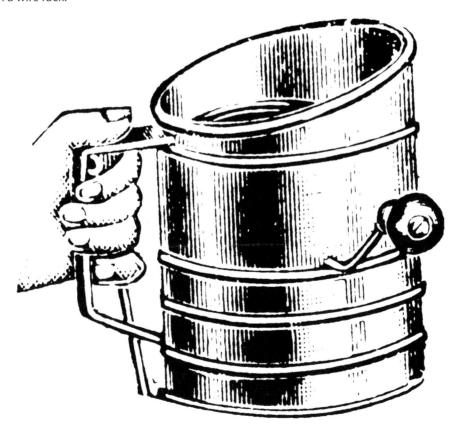

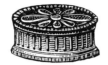

·PATTI PEARSON·

No Bake Chocolate Oatmeal Cookies (Cow Patties)

These are quick and easy and always a hit with the kids. The peanut butter and oats make them less not-healthy, and they have that marvelous carry-around quality that kids enjoy. These work as an after-school/before-practice snack, easily eaten in the car on the way to practice.

2 cups sugar

4 tablespoons cocoa (heaping)

1 stick butter ($^1/_2$ cup)

$^1/_2$ cup milk

$^1/_2$ cup nutty peanut butter

$2^3/_4$ cups quick oats

1 teaspoon vanilla

1. Place sugar, butter, cocoa and milk into saucepan and bring to full boil while stirring. Boil on medium heat 1 minute, stirring constantly so the mixture doesn't burn or stick.
2. Remove from heat and add peanut butter; stir until melted. Add oats and vanilla.
3. Mix thoroughly and drop by teaspoon onto wax paper. Let cool and serve.

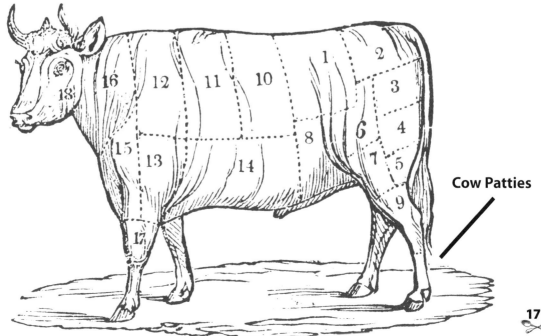

Cow Patties

177

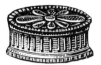
•FRANKIE SEIVERS•

Sugar Cookies

This is a good, old-fashioned recipe, tried and true, a huge favorite with kids and adults alike. Frankie, who is an amazing cook even though she swears she just fixes simple "home-cooking", always gets requests for this recipe when her cookies show up at a potluck. They are simple and delicious; they taste like home. Refrigerating the dough before shaping makes it much easier to handle. This recipe makes a LOT of cookies.

1 cup butter (2 sticks), softened

1 cup vegetable oil

1 cup confectioner's sugar

1 cup sugar

2 teaspoons vanilla

2 eggs, beaten

5 cups flour

1 teaspoon baking soda

1 teaspoon cream of tartar

$^1/_2$ teaspoon salt

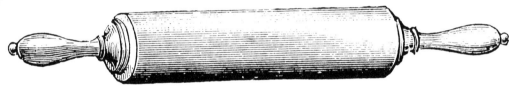

1. Preheat the oven to 350 degrees. Treat a cookie sheet with non-stick spray. Or line a cookie sheet with tinfoil and then treat with non-stick spray. Simply throw away the foil for easy clean-up.
2. Cream butter, oil, the two sugars, vanilla and eggs in a large bowl until light and fluffy.
3. Add flour, soda, cream of tartar, and salt, mixing well. If time allows, refrigerate the dough for at least 2 hours before shaping into cookies; it will be much easier to handle.
4. Shape the dough into small balls and place on an ungreased cookie sheet. Press flat with a glass bottom dipped in sugar.
5. Bake for 10-12 minutes or until light brown around the edges.

Makes 100 cookies

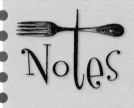

Notes

• *Try adding one teaspoon of lemon extract in exchange for one of the teaspoons of vanilla extract for a subtle change.*
• *Use colored sugar for dipping the glass bottom to celebrate holidays (red for Valentine's Day, pastels for Easter, etc.). Or use your school colors for a team event.*

Pies and Puddings

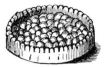

·JEANNE MISENHEIMER·

Peanut Butter Pie

Easy to make, this creamy delight tastes like peanut butter cheesecake. It uses just a few ingredients to produce two mouth-watering pies that will please young and old alike. Teenagers love this one. So do their younger brothers and sisters. If serving at a buffet, be sure to label this one since so many people have peanut allergies.

1 8-ounce package cream cheese (full fat variety), softened

2 cups powdered sugar

1 cup smooth peanut butter

1 cup milk

2 ready-made graham cracker or cookie crumb pie shells

8-ounce container of frozen whipped topping (Cool Whip preferred)

Nuts (optional)

1. Combine the cream cheese and sugar in a mixer. Blend until smooth.
2. Add the peanut butter and milk. Keep blending on medium speed until completely incorporated.
3. Pour into pie shells and top with the whipped topping. Sprinkle with chopped nuts, if using.
4. Refrigerate until ready to serve.

Makes 2 pies

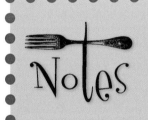

Notes

You could make this in a lower-fat version, using Neufchatel cheese or lower fat cream cheese, low-fat or skim milk, and low-calorie whipped topping. (I'd rather have a small piece of the real deal.)

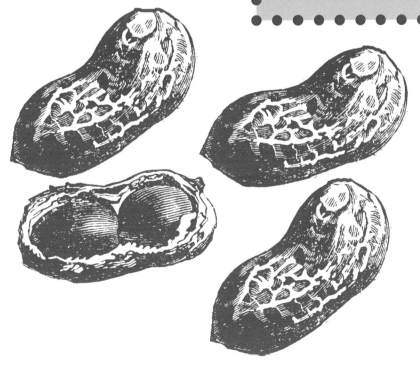

Pies and Puddings

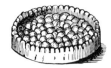

•HELEN WALKER•

Perfect Pumpkin Pie

This is just a fabulous pumpkin pie recipe I got from my Aunt Helen years ago. It is my family's very favorite pie at Thanksgiving. The streusel-like topping brings the power of pecans to the traditional pumpkin flavors. The crunchy texture is sublime against the smoothness of the pumpkin filling. Easy. Fast. Perfect.

FILLING:

1 cup sugar ($^1/_2$ white, $^1/_2$ brown)

3 cups pumpkin puree (2 pints)

1 egg

1 can condensed milk

1 teaspoon cinnamon

$^1/_2$ teaspoon vanilla

Pinch of nutmeg

Optional: lemon zest

Unbaked deep dish pie shell

TOPPING:

1 cup brown sugar

1 cup flour

$^1/_4$ cup butter

$^1/_2$ cup chopped pecans

1. Preheat the oven to 350 degrees.
2. Mix all the filling ingredients well and pour into unbaked pie shell.
3. Pulse the sugar, flour, and butter in a food processor until the mixture resembles cornmeal. Stir in the chopped pecans by hand and spread over the top of the pie.
4. Place the pie plate on a cookie sheet lined with parchment paper or tin foil to catch any drippings if the filling overflows during baking.
5. Bake for 55 minutes.

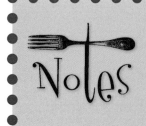

Notes

I like to use frozen pie shells that come in sets of two for this recipe. The filling is a bit too much for just one pie shell, so I use the extra crust for the remaining filling.

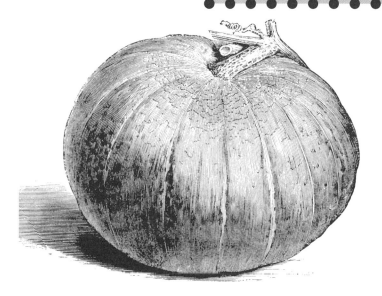

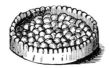
·FRANKIE SEIVERS·

Bread Pudding With Spiced Rum Sauce

The flavors of this wonderful recipe are simple and old fashioned: sweet bread custard spiced with raisins, cinnamon and rum. It is the perfect make-ahead dish since it requires soaking overnight. If you don't want real rum in the sauce, just leave it out and add a teaspoon of rum flavoring. Or just eliminate the rum presence altogether.

PUDDING:

8 large eggs

3^1/$_2$ cups whole milk

2 cups sugar

^{1}/$_2$ cup whipping cream

1 teaspoon vanilla

1 loaf French bread, cut into 1" cubes

1 cup golden raisins

1. Butter a 13x9x2-inch glass dish.
2. Whisk eggs in a large bowl to blend.
3. Add milk, sugar, cream and vanilla. Whisk to blend well.
4. Stir in bread and raisins; pour mixture into buttered dish; cover and refrigerate overnight.
5. Preheat the oven to 350 degrees. Bake the pudding uncovered until puffed and golden, about 1^1/$_4$ hours. Serve with Spiced Rum Sauce.

SPICED RUM SAUCE:

1 cup dark brown sugar, packed

^{1}/$_2$ cup (1 stick) unsalted butter

^{1}/$_2$ cup heavy whipping cream

2 tablespoons dark rum or spiced rum

1 teaspoon ground cinnamon

1. Stir brown sugar and butter in a heavy medium sauce pan over medium heat until melted and smooth, about 2 minutes
2. Add cream, rum and cinnamon; bring to a simmer. Simmer until sauce thickens and reduces to 1^1/$_2$ cups (about 5 minutes.)
3. Serve warm over bread pudding.

Serves 6-8

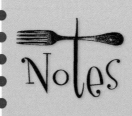

Notes

• *Stale bread is essential for this recipe to work. Fresh bread has too much moisture and produces a mushy result. If the bread is fresh, cut it up the night before and let it sit out in the air overnight. (Yes!)*

• *Bourbon could be substituted for the rum if that is what you have on your shelf.*

• *You could use regular raisins instead of golden raisins – still delicious!*

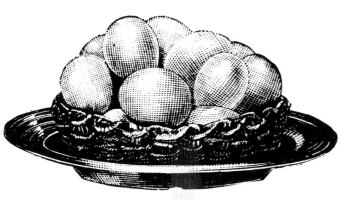

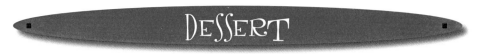

DESSERT

Fruit

•FRANKIE SEIVERS•

Apple Pockets

These are tasty little apple turnovers without the fuss. They are perfect individual servings and would be great on a fall menu. As a dessert, they would nicely balance a menu short on fresh fruits or vegetables (like spaghetti or Stromboli, for example). Serve warm with a dollop of vanilla ice cream.

2 cans of refrigerated crescent rolls

2 tart apples, each peeled and cut into eight pieces (Granny Smith are perfect)

1 cup sugar

1 cup water

$^1/_2$ stick butter (4 tablespoons)

Cinnamon

1. Preheat the oven to 325 degrees. Prepare a roasting pan or baking sheet with high sides with non-stick spray, or use a non-stick mat like Silpat.
2. Open the rolls and separate the dough into pre-cut triangles.
3. Starting at the large end, roll each piece of apple in a triangle. Pinch the ends closed.
4. Boil together the water, sugar and butter. Set aside to cool.
5. Settle the apples in the prepared pan, leaving room in between each for the dough to expand. Pour the sugar mixture over the apples; sprinkle with cinnamon.
6. Bake 30 minutes, until the dough is golden and the apples are softened.

16 individual servings

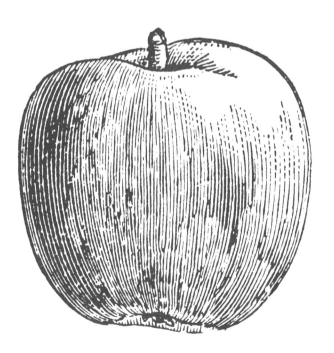

Fruit

No-Fuss Peach Cobbler

I've used this recipe many years. I got it from a wonderful cook who worked with my husband and who always brought the tastiest dishes to office parties. It has been around a long time – note the unmodern high fat and sugar content. Nothing beats hot peaches covered with a moist sweet biscuit topping. It is so good, and so easy to make. Even though the peaches are layered in last, they end up on the bottom. You could use a number of fruits in place of the peaches, but fresh peaches are my favorite.

$^1/_4$ **cup plus 2 tablespoons butter**

2 cups sugar, divided

$^3/_4$ **cup all-purpose flour (will have salt and leavening added)**

2 teaspoons baking powder

Dash of salt

$^3/_4$ **cups milk**

2 cups peeled, sliced peaches

Vanilla ice cream or whipped cream optional

1. Preheat the oven to 350 degrees. You do not need to pre-treat a casserole.
2. Melt butter in a 2 quart baking dish.
3. Combine 1 cup sugar, flour, baking powder and salt; add milk and stir until mixed.
4. Pour batter evenly over butter in baking dish, but do not stir.
5. Combine peaches and remaining 1 cup of sugar; spoon over the batter. Do not stir.
6. Bake for 1 hour, until puffy and golden. Serve warm with ice cream.

Yield: 6-8 servings

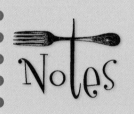

Notes

• I find this makes a very rich cobbler. I cut down the amount of butter by the extra two tablespoons and it works fine.
• This recipe is also very sweet. I would start by adding about $^1/_4$ cup sugar to the peaches and then taste as you go. Depending on the ripeness of the peaches, you may need much less sugar than the recipe calls for. Unless you just want your teeth to hurt.
• Remember, you can serve this in whatever you bake it, so pick a pretty pan.
• IF there is any left over, it can be microwaved briefly before serving again so the ice cream melts.

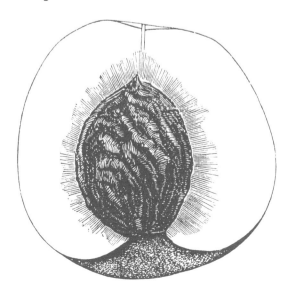

Fruit

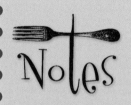

Sensational Strawberries

This is a classic preparation for strawberries. They taste like they have been dipped in caramel. The tart sour cream and crunchy brown sugar are an incredible compliment to the fresh, smooth taste of the berry. Simple and impressive, this makes a great yet easy dessert. You can dip the berries for your guests, or put out a bowl of sour cream and brown sugar and let them dip for themselves, like a fondue. It is a fun dessert for teens, especially the ones who don't want a fattening finish to meals, but still crave a little sweet. It's a great way to get kids to eat their fruit, too!

Strawberries, cleaned and hulled

Sour cream

Brown sugar

Fresh mint for garnish

1. Dip a berry in the sour cream and then roll it in the brown sugar. Sprinkle with finely chopped mint, if using.
2. Eat.

Notes

• *The ratio of sour cream to sugar is a matter of personal preference. You can go heavy on the sour cream and light on the sugar for a tarter taste, or roll that berry in the sugar until it is almost too heavy to pick it up!*

• *This is a great treatment for berries that aren't prime and sweet – you'll never know by the time you finish rolling them around in the sour cream and sugar.*

• *You can leave the green cap on the strawberry as a handle if you want to serve informally and let everyone dip their own– just be sure to put out a bowl to catch the caps.*

• *This is a pretty presentation served on a long rectangular serving platter. Garnish with sprigs of fresh mint at the edges or chop it finely and sprinkle over the platter of berries. Mint adds a refreshing little hit in the midst of all that sweetness.*

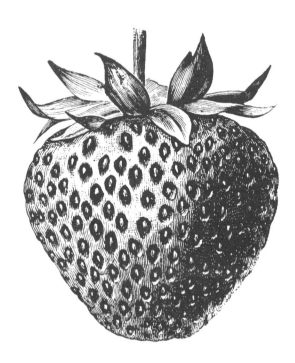

Fruit

Strawberry Surprise

I remember my mom fixing this as I was growing up. She always served it as party food, but never failed to save some for the kids because she knew how much we loved it. This is an unusual recipe. The crust is chewy on the inside, almost like toffee. The fruit and whipped cream topping is good by itself, but combined with the nutty, chewy crust, it becomes something more than the sum of its parts. This is a perfect spring dessert for a ladies' lunch.

CRUST:

3 egg whites, room temperature

1 cup sugar

Pinch of salt

1 teaspoon baking powder

1 teaspoon vanilla

1 cup pecans, toasted and chopped

24 Ritz crackers, crushed

TOPPING:

1 pint whipping cream

1 tablespoon sugar

¹/₂ cup crushed pineapple

Fresh strawberries

Fresh mint leaves (optional)

1. Preheat the oven to 325 degrees. Treat a pie plate or low-sided pan with non-stick spray.
2. Beat egg whites until stiff in a large bowl (see note below). Gradually add the sugar until it is all incorporated. Be careful to not overbeat the sugar and whites – you don't want a glossy stiff meringue, just sweet whites with good body. Then add a pinch of salt and the baking powder.
3. Stir in vanilla.
4. Fold in nuts and crackers. Spoon into the prepared pie plate or pan. Even out the mixture with the back of a tablespoon.
5. Bake for 35-40 minutes until golden; cool and refrigerate.
6. When you are ready to serve, whip the cream (see note), being careful not to overbeat; you have gone too far if the cream starts to get chunky. As soon as you can run a finger through the cream and it doesn't fold onto itself but holds its shape around the ditch you made with your finger, stop whipping. Fold in sugar, pineapple, and strawberries carefully.
7. To serve: cut a wedge of crust and top with a dollop of fruit mixture. Or spread the fruit and cream on top of the crust and cut like a pie. Garnish with a small, perfect berry and a sprig of mint.

Serves 6-8

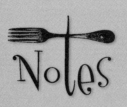

Notes

- Take a minute or two to toast the pecans – don't skip this step. You can bake them in a 400 degree oven for about 7-8 minutes, watching them carefully to prevent burning. Or toss them in a skillet on medium high heat until they toast, around 5 minutes. They will burn quickly once they get hot, so don't leave them unattended.
- To crush the crackers, place them in a zip top bag and pound them with the side of a rolling pin.
- Of course you could use frozen dessert topping, but the richness and luxury of real whipped cream elevates this simple dessert. To get the most out of your whipping cream, place the beaters and bowl in the freezer for a few minutes before you whip the cream. The colder, the better. You don't need a huge bowl to whip cream; it doesn't incorporate as much air as the egg whites do.
- To beat egg whites: make sure the whites are at room temperature. Use a large bowl since the idea behind whipping the whites is to incorporate as much air as possible. Also, be sure your beaters are spotlessly clean. Even the smallest amount of grease or oil will inhibit the expansion process. If any of the yolk gets caught in the white when you separate the egg, it will keep the whites from fully expanding.

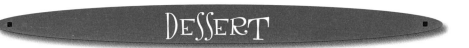

Snacks

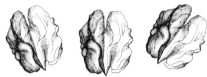

•CINDY BAIRD•
Fun-To-Make Cereal Mix

Kids love to make this one themselves. And they love to eat it, too. It has some healthy-ish ingredients, so you don't have to stand over them and ration it out. Fix up zip top bags of this for an after-school snack, or snack before practice, or on the bus ride to a game.

1 package + 3 squares of almond bark

1 box Crispix cereal

$^1/_2$ bag of stick pretzels

1 pound package of plain M&M's

1 12-ounce can of salted peanuts

1. Melt bark in microwave according to package directions.
2. Mix the cereal, pretzels, M&M's, and peanuts in a bowl. Pour the melted bark over mix and stir well. Spread on a piece of wax paper to cool.
3. Break into pieces and store in an airtight container.

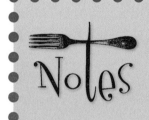
Notes

There are no notes. Of course, you could vary the candy if your kids don't like M&M's. You could use raisins, almonds, dried fruit – but why mess with perfection?

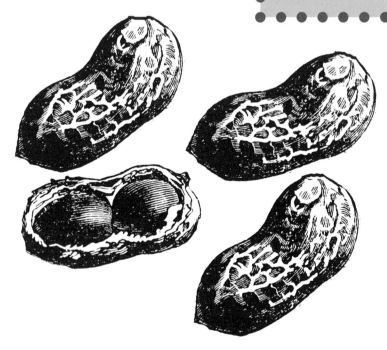

Snacks

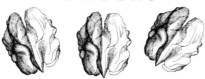

•PATTI PEARSON•

Nutty Cereal Snack

Here is one of those cereal snacks the kids love – plus it can be color coordinated to the season. It goes together quickly and can be served individually or in a big, festive bowl. This makes a great after-school snack or treat for the bus ride to or from a game. The kids can get involved in making this one – just be careful with the hot syrup.

12-ounce package square bite size rice cereal (12 cups)

12-ounce package M&M's (1^1/$_2$ cups)

2-ounce package slivered almonds

3.75-ounce package shelled sunflower seeds

1 cup (2 sticks) plus 2 tablespoons margarine or butter

1^1/$_2$ cups sugar

1^1/$_2$ cups light corn syrup

1^1/$_2$ teaspoons vanilla

1. In a very large container combine cereal, M&M's, almonds and sunflower seeds. Set aside.
2. In a large saucepan, melt butter. Add sugar and syrup to a non-stick saucepan and stir to combine. Bring mixture to a boil over medium heat. Boil gently for 3 minutes while stirring frequently so it doesn't stick or burn. Remove pan from heat and stir in vanilla.
3. Pour syrup over cereal mixture while stirring, until pieces are coated. Turn out onto waxed paper.
4. Let stand, covered with waxed paper, for several hours or overnight.
5. Break into clusters. Wrap clusters in plastic wrap or serve in a large bowl.

Makes 20 cups

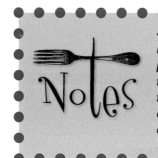

Notes

• *Make this a seasonal treat by using different colored M&M's: pastel for Easter, red and green for Christmas; black and orange for Halloween, etc. You could even tint the syrup with a few drops of food coloring.*

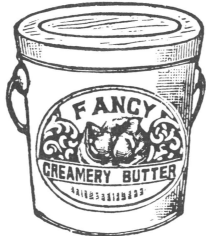

FANCY CREAMERY BUTTER

	• Single Serving	• 12 guests	• 25 guests
BREAD			
Rolls or muffins	1$\frac{1}{2}$	18-24	3$\frac{1}{2}$ dozen
DESSERT			
Ice cream	6 ounces	2 quarts	1 gallon
Layer cake	1 slice	1 8-inch cake	2 8-inch cakes
Sheet cake	2x2-inch piece	less than $\frac{1}{4}$ sheet	$\frac{1}{4}$ sheet
Brownies/bars	1-2	16-18	2$\frac{1}{2}$-3 dozen
Cookies	2-3	3-4 dozen	6-8 dozen

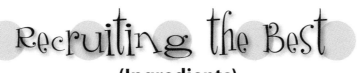

Recruiting the Best
(Ingredients)

EXCEPTIONAL INGREDIENTS make exceptional dishes, no matter how simple the procedure. It is easy to locate outstanding or unusual ingredients with the help of the Internet. In fact, the easiest way to locate an ingredient is to "Google" it. Just go to google.com and type in your ingredient. You will find a slew of websites to suit your needs. You may also discover fabulous recipes at some of these websites. I find that the recipes included on the back of a package or at the home website for a product are often quite good, since they are designed to showcase the product and you can be sure they have been well-tested.

Most of the ingredients you will need for the recipes in this book are readily available at the supermarket or gourmet store. But you may want to walk on the wild side every once in a while and try a new ingredient or search out the best of the best of a simple thing like cinnamon or pasta. Here are some of my favorite sites for procuring exceptional quality and variety in ingredients.

• A.G. Ferrari Brothers - www.agferrari.com - *Italian ingredients*
This wonderful grocery, with locations in northern California, sells its remarkable ingredients online. The dried pasta is truly exceptional, and the sauces are the freshest-tasting I have encountered in a jar. The owners make several trips to Italy each year, searching out small, artisanal producers of cheese, oil, jams, pasta, sauces, cakes, truffles, and meats. The easy-to-use site includes recipes, and it groups products by both type and region. My family can tell the difference when I use these ingredients. If Ferrari sells it, it's good. Be sure to splurge at least once on the Makaira Spaghetti all Chitarra. It will be hard to go back to any other spaghetti product. Fabulous.

• D'artagnan - www.dartagnan - *Gourmet meat and game, truffles, foie gras*
This wonderful site carries the fancy stuff and has recipes to help you use it. Wagyu beef, truffle oil, demi-glace – it's all here. You can sign up for a newsletter that is full of specials and recipes. You don't even have to use the products. You can learn a lot just reading their website and e-mails.

• Ethnic Grocer - www.ethnicgrocer.com - *Ethnic spices and ingredients*
This virtual grocery store makes cooking anything ethnic a breeze. In addition to ingredients classified by country, it includes recipes that use the exotic stuff for sale. A fun site to explore.

• Penzey's Spices - www.penzeys.com - *Fresh spices*
This company, my all-time favorite spice source, sells more spices than I knew existed. In addition to having every individual spice under the sun, including numerous cinnamons and peppercorns, it also makes proprietary blends of seasonings for salads, pasta, grilling – you name it. I have tried a large majority of them, and have been impressed with the quality, freshness, and inventiveness of the combinations. Two of my favorites, the Chip and Dip seasoning, and Italian dressing seasoning, I keep on hand all the time. The site has some great recipes on file, too. Sign up for their catalog; it has great ideas and recipes. You can learn a lot about each spice from reading the descriptions.

• The Rosengarten Report – www.Davidrosengarten.com - *mail-order food, wine, travel*
David Rosengarten writes a monthly newsletter about the best food and wine available by mail or phone. He evaluates a huge number of products, selects the best and tells you how to get it, since it might not have been discovered yet by your local gourmet store. Sometimes his supplier is a restaurant that only sells directly to the public. He wrote the Dean and DeLuca cookbook and has devoted his life to tasting and writing about food. You can trust his palate. His newsletter is a treasure of sources for food, wine, and travel experiences. It is a fun, mouth-watering read. He also has an olive oil club that is well worth the money if you enjoy the nuances of the flavors of olive oil.

• Virtual Cajun - www.virtualcajun.com – *Cajun ingredients*
This website has plenty of interesting selections for condiments and spices for preparing Cajun dishes, but my favorite item is Kary's roux in a jar. This convenience makes gumbo a lot easier to prepare. It also carries Slap Ya Mama seasoning (a mix of salt, various peppers and garlic) and Boudreaux Butt Paste (an anti-itch cream), two items I want to buy for the name alone.

• Cajun Wholesale – www. Cajunwholesale.com – *Cajun ingredients*
This fun site has the expected fiery, flavorful seasonings as well as Cajun music, grills, aprons, gift packs, Mardi Gras beads and cookbooks. My favorite item is the jar of Cajun Power Sloppy Boudreaux (Sloppy Joes to the rest of us.)

• Zingerman's - www.zingermans.com - *cheese, olive oil, bread, baked goods, meat, condiments*
This is one of my favorite places to browse on-line. It is a foodie's paradise. I have ordered many times and always been delighted. The array of freshly baked breads (the pepper-Parmesan – oh my), cakes and brownies is tempting, but the choice of cheeses, meats, coffee, and oils and vinegars is really quite excellent. You can't go wrong with something from Zingerman's. They have great gift baskets, too. They aren't cheap, but they are worth it.

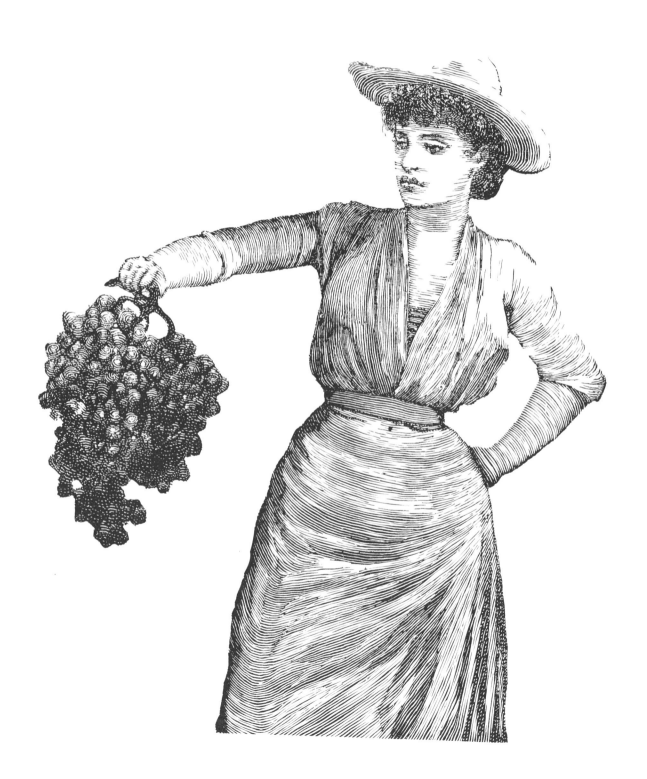

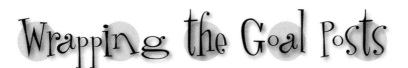

Wrapping the Goal Posts

Transforming the Venue

DECORATING FOR A SCHOOL or athletic event may be your idea of hell. I shopped on that aisle for many years. Then I met some extremely creative women who showed me the path to enlightenment. They convinced me that establishing a theme was the critical factor in decorating serenity.

If you have a theme, many of your choices become obvious, from the menu to the decorating. An Italian night, a Southern Comfort meal, a "Beat the Dawgs" blast – each of these themes suggests ideas not only for the food, but the decorations, too, from color scheme to centerpieces. Don't underestimate the effect that simple decorations can have on an event; they make the moment feel festive, and they make the participants feel special. Decorations, even without being elaborate, can make a simple meal feel like a party. And everyone loves a party!

Let's look at how the simple decision to use "Breakfast for Lunch" as a theme could make the menu and decoration decisions – if not easy, then at least a little more obvious.

Serve breakfast favorites like waffles (maybe a dress-your-own waffle bar?), bacon, sausage and biscuits, cut fruit or fruit juice, and sweet rolls. Stuffed animals from home could be recruited as adorable table decorations. Complement them with a pastel color theme. Inexpensive baby blankets would make great table toppers. You could even roll out sleeping bags around the room, or have piles of pillows, slippers and stuffed animals arranged semi-artfully in a corner to set the stage. None of this requires a lot of money, but the kids will enjoy it.

Decorating the eating space for kids is actually sort of fun. It's important to remember—you are decorating for kids! They are not impressed with expensive fabrics, elaborate staging, and intricate doo-dads. They aren't going to care if you got your materials from an interior design store or the dollar store. They won't notice if the flowers on a table are orchids or carnations.

Kids notice the big stuff: balloons, colorful signs, streamers, buckets of candy. One of the best decorating ideas I've seen is buying large bags of inexpensive, individually wrapped candy from a food club store and scattering the goodies on the kids' tables. They go wild. They remember the candy and talk about it for days. A lot of bang for very little buck. You can even coordinate your candy to the theme: hot tamales for a Mexican fiesta, Baby Ruth's for a baseball event, wrappers that use the school or team colors. You now have a legitimate reason to linger on the candy aisle, scoping out the decorating options. (At least that's your story, if anyone asks.)

Another affordable and enjoyable decorating idea is to take lots of pictures of the kids and display them. Kids are crazy about looking at each other's pictures at any age. For our Senior Lunches, which were done 5 times during the school year, we started taking pictures of the kids and parents right off the bat at the first four lunches. By the time we got to the last, bittersweet lunch, we had a stack of pictures. We taped a piece of butcher paper to the wall for each of the four previous meals and attached the appropriate pictures taken from each event. The kids had a great time traveling around the room, looking at the pictures from each month, and reliving the year. If you are organized enough, you could have one person in charge of photography who keeps all the photos on file digitally. A CD of all the prints could be made as parting gifts for the seniors, assuming you don't have 2,000 in your graduating class.

This concept works well for team events, too. Have a collection of photos taken of the team during games, on bus rides, etc. through the years, and hand them down each year to the team parent. Then, at the first parent's meeting, display those pictures on good old butcher paper hung on a wall. I guarantee they will be a hit, and your decorations will be halfway done!

Another caveat of decorating for kids is having as many helping hands as possible; don't try to do it all by yourself. Decide on your theme early and then brainstorm. Multiple heads are always better than one, as long as you have a clear leader. Start your planning early so you can have all the ingredients on hand. If you are decorating an event for older kids, include them in your planning. They come up with some great ideas, and they bring enthusiasm and extra hands to the venture.

Check out any parental connections your class or team might have. Someone may work with a food chain or restaurant, at a plant nursery, or with a paper or party supply store. See if they can get either an employee discount or a great "school deal." Some stores (we have had great experiences with TCBY frozen yogurt and Subway sandwich shops) may have a discounted price for schools, even without the parental connection. Ask! You might even develop a working relationship with a restaurant and use them as your go-to source for team meals or parties – something you could make clear early in the conversation.

I've had the good fortune to work with some very talented, creative women through the years. My squad of decorating experts (all of whom have beautiful homes, beautiful children, or both!) helped me devise a list of cheap, showy materials and great ideas that you can use to create a festive atmosphere.

• Forget the glamour – go for the **cheap plastic tablecloths**! They come in a huge array of colors and sizes. They can be cut on-site to fit the table. They can even be used to wrap leftover wet stuff if you are truly desperate. You might even be able to use them again. You can also buy the colored table cloth plastic on big rolls if you are covering a lot of tables or have some really long table spans. Check with party supply stores or paper/stationary outlets. Keep an eye out for sales.

• A wonderful, funky alternative to the plastic tablecloth is a **great big roll of brown paper**. The advantage here is you don't have a lot of hang-down on the table side - highly desirable if you are feeding young, squirmy kids and don't want table-cloths that pull off easily. Also, the kids can draw on them. Pass out crayons and let them go to town while they wait for the meeting to finish or for a parent to bring a plateful of food. Just tape the paper to the underside of the table. White butcher paper can be used the same way.

• If you want to add some pizzazz to the table, layer colored cellophane - available in rolls - over your plastic or paper base. After-Easter sales are a good time to stock up.

• To achieve a finished look at the corners of the table that perhaps hides hastily taped paper or plastic, **add large bows**. You can make them from Mylar, floral ribbon, wide tulle, cellophane, or faux raffia. Make plenty of bows and scatter them around the room in appropriate areas to get a unified look (to look like they are holding up signs? At the registration table? Somewhere on the centerpiece? At the bottom of a balloon cluster?)

• To give flower containers used at a lot of tables a uniform look, wrap them with colored tissue paper and tie with faux raffia or ribbons. You can use almost any inexpensive container, like terra cotta pots or empty cans, and fluff them up with tissue. Set the container in the center of several sheets of tissue paper and pull the tissue straight up. Tie a ribbon around the circumference of the container to hold the paper in place, then pretty up the edges, either cutting them down to the appropriate length or spreading them out. Get that color scheme working here.

• Brown lunch bags can be used a hundred different ways, and they are wildly inexpensive. Cover a potted plant with a bag and then tie it with ribbons and bows. Roll down the top a bit and fill it with unshelled peanuts. Or candy. Place several on each table. If you are using them for bagged lunches for a team, take just a little bit of time and draw a quick decoration on it with magic markers - maybe the team name or logo, a player's number, a feisty saying (Go Groundhogs!), or a season-appropriate saying. If you are providing bag lunches for the visiting team between games, resist the urge to write trash talk on the bags.

• If you need arrangements for a lot of tables, consider **contacting a nursery** and either borrowing some potted plants that will be returned without fail the next morning (this works best if you have a parent connection to the nursery), or sell the potted plants at the end of dinner as a fund-raiser for the team. Mums and poinsettias are great for this. See if you can buy them at a bulk rate or if the nursery will give you a "school rate" to help with your profit. Offer them free advertising in the school newspaper or yearbook as an incentive. Also, be sure to acknowledge their contribution during the event in the program or with little signs on the tables.

• **Terra cotta pots** are cheap and can be painted to suit any theme or color scheme. Tie a ribbon or raffia around them for added fluff. Use them for silverware, napkins, straws, condiments, flowers, candy, pencils, and name tags – anything that needs holding. Colored polka dots make a cute decoration that is easy to draw and general enough to be used in a variety of settings (girls/ boys/ teams/ teachers etc.) Pots painted in school colors can be stored and used again from year to year. Cute stuff can also be glued on for quick décor; buttons are good. Some other embellishments: fun colored or shaped pasta (Italian night, maybe?); fake jewels; anything from the craft store that comes in a big bag like googley eyes, those fluffy little balls, beads; mirror or mosaic pieces; stickers. Check the scrapbooking areas. Hot glue grosgrain ribbon in criss-cross patterns or stripes in school or team colors.

• **Butcher paper** can be transformed in so many ways. Hang a big sheet on the cafeteria wall and fill it with snapshots of the kids. Or let the kids sign a banner for Teacher Appreciation Day – lay it out on the sidewalk and let them all write something and then hang it in the celebration room. Or slap it on a table for a quick tablecloth. Use it to wrap the bottom of a stage or hide ugly legs on risers. And of course, use it to make signs (or rather, have the cheerleaders make signs. . .)

• **Incorporate sports equipment** into your decorating for sports events. Caps and shoes make whimsical containers for flower arrangements on the buffet table. Grouping items together on the table or floor adds impact. Just make sure it doesn't end up looking like your son's chaotic bedroom at the end of the season. . .

• Balloons are a staple at almost any school or team function. They add instant impact, lots of color, they are pretty cheap – and the kids love sucking the helium out of them. Use them weighted down to mark important locations. Tie them to the back of a chair. Wrap their tails around a brick and use them as a centerpiece. Make a pile of bats or other sports equipment decorative by tying balloons to them. Attach them to signs. Use them at the entrance to the room. Mark the tailgate vehicle with a bunch attached to the side mirror or the antenna, especially if you have a lovely "vintage" car. Balloons are life's confetti – they lend an air of festivity to anything you do with kids.

• The all-time kid-favored balloon decoration – unfortunately – is the traditional balloon arch. It can be made for homecoming or special events, but it requires a bit of planning and the more hands, the better. You will need to rent one or two large canisters of helium. Use a string to measure the length of your arch. Lay it out on the ground to figure out how much length you will need. You can tie the balloons to the measuring string or to sturdy fishing line – the line isn't going to show, so it doesn't matter. It helps to suspend the string up off the ground while you are tying on the (millions of) balloons. Tie the string between bleachers or the backs of chairs. This one is a pain to do, but the result is spectacular. The football team loves running through the balloon arch at Homecoming games.

• Put out signs on the school campus to advertise your event. Real estate signs can be covered with poster board. Staple two pieces of board together and slip it over the sign. Punch holes in the corners and attach balloons tied with ribbons.

• **Become familiar with what is available** at the different supply stores. When you know your raw materials, you can get more creative. Keep a lookout for seasonal things that go on sale and stock up for the next year, from candles, paper, ribbons and trim, to paper cups, plates and cutlery. You might get lucky and find serving pieces in sports shapes or school colors greatly reduced. Pass them on when your kids graduate.

The holidays usually arrive with a full calendar of parties and events. If you have to spruce up an eating area for one of these parties, try some of these Christmas ideas:

• Wrap the dining table like a great big present. Cover the table with solid or printed paper (use the rolls of colored plastic tablecloths available at party supply stores) and tape the edges under. Run bands of ribbon in a cross shape across the top and tape under at the edges of the table. Tie a great big bow made with wide ribbon and secure it in the center of the table. Voila! Table cloth and centerpiece: DONE.

• Wrap empty boxes with inexpensive wrapping paper and bows and pile them around as random decorations in a corner or place on the table as a centerpiece.

• Oversized pieces of candy make a fun decoration, a lot of bang for the buck. To make: wrap a paper towel tube with pretty paper and tie the ends like an English cracker treat. Stripe paper plates with red magic marker. Glue two together, insides facing each other, and wrap with clear cellophane leaving extra at each end. Twist the ends and tie with ribbon. So cute! So easy!

• If your event is one or two days before Christmas, wait until the last minute to buy some fresh-cut trees. You can sometimes get them at a big discount late in the season.

• If you are the head decorating honcho, it always helps to have a go-to basket full of miscellaneous stuff that usually gets used:
    • scotch and masking tape
    • scissors
    • magic markers and Sharpies
    • extra pens and pencils; notebook paper
    • rubber bands
    • thumb tacks
    • hammer and screw driver
    • the phone numbers of school personnel and main committee people involved with the project
    • twist ties (you'd be surprised)
    • a few garbage bags
    • Throw in a camera to record the proceedings – you're making decorations for next year!

Roster of Contributors

Cindy Baird – mother of five, veteran team mom, volunteer organizer; Knoxville, TN

Sheron Bibee – mother and proud grandmother, epitome of school volunteer/ team/ room mom; Knoxville, TN

Mary Constantine – food writer for the Knoxville News Sentinel; Knoxville, TN

Linda Deaver – mom and cooking enthusiast; Knoxville, TN

Mary Faircloth – co-author of Crispy Parmesan Toasts; Grand Forks, ND

Mike Fields – cook, Flat Creek Ranch; Jackson Hole, WY

Leslie Gallaher – retired teacher, ardent Tennessee Vols fan and tailgater, intrepid sailor; Knoxville, TN

Helen Georgi - mother and elegant entertainer – a true southern lady and dear family friend; Memphis, TN

Kathy Hall – event planner, fashion coordinator (and just plain elegant); Knoxville, TN

Ruby Herring – mom (mine) of four and doting grandmother, experimental cook extraordinaire; Memphis, TN

Sharon Herring – site locator for films; California-healthy food sensibilities; Hermosa Beach, CA

Missy Hutton – team cook, mom, and food organizer for Loudon county school; Lenoir City, TN

Shirley Jarvis – mother of four and grandmother; one of the best cooks I know; Johnson City, TN

Jackie Jarvis Jones – one in a family of exceptional cooks, attorney and mom of two; Charlotte, NC

Joan Jordan – church potluck veteran and workout buddy; Marshall, AK

Tillie Lungaro – mom of four and adoring grandmother, elegant entertainer for Mardi Gras Crewe; Lake Charles, LA

Cathy Mellot – Fly fisherman and long-time community cook; New Enterprise, PA

Jeanne Misenheimer – mom of two, teacher and school administrator, baseball mom; Knoxville, TN

Leah Moir – "everybody's mom", church and elementary school food services director; Knoxville, TN

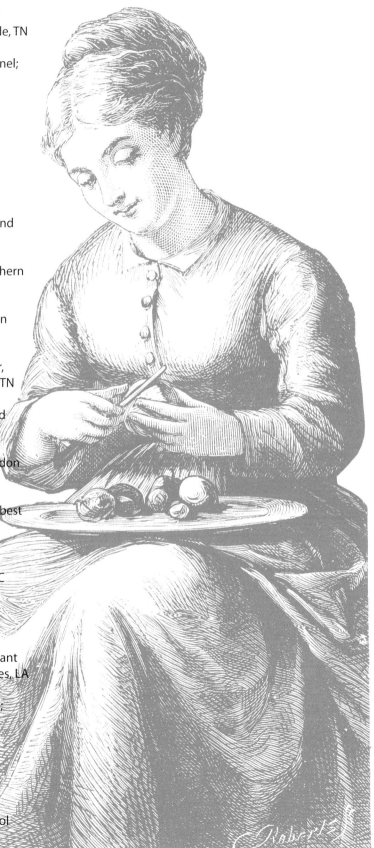

John Mullaney – associate pastor, Vestavia Hills Methodist Church, Birmingham, AL

Pam Mullins – horse-show judge, host of countless dinner parties; Collierville, TN and Wellington, FL

Patti Pearson – mom of two; volunteer event organizer and decorator; makes any venue look fabulous; Knoxville, TN

Susan Porter Levy – mother of adored Rachel, psycho-neurobiologist with finely-tuned spiritual and health sensibilities; McKinney, TX

Len Pousson – mom of four; model; camping veteran; Lake Charles, LA

Carol Powell – ultrasound technician and former special education teacher; amateur chicken raiser and sometime gardener, transplanted city girl who's happily turned hillbilly; Pottersville, MO

Jeanette Reisenburg – university administrator and city council member, Laramie, Wyoming; cook, host, and guide at high camp at Flat Creek Ranch, Jackson Hole, Wyoming

Diane Robbins – mom and grandmother, experienced hostess with a finely develop palate; Helena, AK

Maureen Rowan – "the cookie lady", cooking entrepreneur and real estate agent, workout buddy; Knoxville, TN

Frankie Seivers – mother of University of Tennessee Hall of Fame Receiver, Larry Seivers; grandmother; ardent sports fan; everyone's favorite potluck contributor; Clinton, TN

Helen Walker – mom of three and grandmother; host and cook for endless family gatherings; Lake Charles, LA

Webb Friday Night Feasts – informal handbook of recipes for the high school football team of Webb School of Knoxville, compiled by moms through the years; Knoxville, TN

Index

Index

Index

Index

Index